The Cancer Connection

And What We Can Do about It

The Cancer Connection

And What We Can Do about It

by Larry Agran

Houghton Mifflin Company · Boston · 1977

Library of Congress Cataloging in Publication Data

Agran, Larry.
  The cancer connection.

  Bibliography: p.
  Includes index.
  1. Cancer—Prevention.   2. Carcinogens.
3. Occupational diseases.   4. Environmentally induced
diseases.   I. Title.
RC268.A37   616.9'94'05   76-58920
ISBN 0-395-25178-8

Printed in the United States of America
00 10 9 8 7 6 5 4 3 2 1

Brief portions of chapters one and two appeared in slightly
different form in an article, "Getting Cancer on the Job," by
Larry Agran, in *The Nation*, April 12, 1975.

"Take My Hand, Precious Lord" by Thomas A. Dorsey
Copyright © 1938 by Hill and Range Songs, Inc.
Copyright Renewed, assigned to Unichappell Music, Inc.
International Copyright Secured. All rights reserved.
Used by permission.
  Dr. Alton Ochsner's recollections, quoted on pages 118
and 121, are reprinted with the kind permission of Dr. Ernst
Wynder, President of the American Health Foundation. Dr.
Ochsner's article, "Corner of History: My First Recognition
of the Relationship of Smoking and Lung Cancer,"
appeared in *Preventive Medicine*, Vol. 2, 1973, pp. 611–614.

To those holding positions of high authority . . .

That they might See the cancer pox, Understand its origins, and Act to reverse its deadly momentum.

Author's Note

I HAVE NOT WISHED to burden the text with distracting foot-
notes. However, believing as I do that documentation is important in a work of this nature, I have included a section of notes and
sources of information, arranged by chapter and page.

Acknowledgments

IN 1974, CAREY MCWILLIAMS, who was then the editor of *The Nation,* was instrumental in arranging for a travel grant to further my investigative work which, at that time, focused chiefly on the problems of occupationally caused cancers. I was grateful then, as I am now, for the early support that he provided.

Throughout 1975 and 1976, as my investigation into national cancer policies broadened, the list of those who lent assistance began to lengthen. Drs. Reuben Merliss, Rea Schneider, Delmar Pascoe, and Arthur Ablin contacted cancer victims on my behalf, asking that they avail themselves for the in-depth interviews that are now an integral part of this book. Dr. Michael Shimkin facilitated my preparation of Chapters 7 and 8 by loaning his collection of early cigarette advertisements.

While parts of this book have passed before many eyes on its way into print, I am particularly indebted to three individuals who so conscientiously reviewed and criticized the entire manuscript: Dr. Hector Blejer, Professor Lawrence J. Friedman, and Dr. Wilhelm C. Hueper.

I am appreciative of Ellen Joseph's editorial contributions to this book. Over a period spanning many months, her editing was consistently skillful and always characterized by a judicious blend of criticism and encouragement.

In addition to those already mentioned, there are scores of government officials — at this juncture they are best left nameless — who provided information essential to documenting the nature and course of America's cancer epidemic. Their cooperation and their concern reinforce my belief that a traditional spirit of public service still resides among countless government employees. What we have lacked is effective leadership at the highest levels to draw upon this reservoir of talent and dedication.

Finally, I owe a special note of thanks to the individuals — and their relatives — who granted me lengthy interviews to document the human dimensions of the cancer pox. At the time of our interviews, several of these people surely sensed that they would not live to see their own words in print. But in each case they went ahead, expressing the hope that in recounting their own experiences they might contribute to public policies designed to prevent future cancer tragedies. We shared that common objective. And, indeed, that is the purpose of this book.

Preface

APRIL 12, 1955. A MILESTONE IN THE CHRONICLE OF HUMAN HISTORY. It was on that Tuesday that Dr. Jonas Salk announced to the American public, and to the entire world, that he had developed a successful vaccine against the crippling viral disease, poliomyelitis. In a matter of months, millions of Americans, children and adults, were immunized against polio. Within a few years the wondrous antipolio vaccine had been so thoroughly distributed across the country that we quickly forgot how it used to be. When summers were known as "the polio season." When public swimming pools were closed. When fearful parents cautioned their children to avoid crowds. By the early 1960's all that was gone. Gone, too, was the looming horror of children with lifeless limbs, caged in iron lungs. Vanquished by the genius of modern medical science, polio was no longer a significant factor in American life.

Understandably, the conquest of polio provided the American people with added confidence that another crippler and killer, the most frightful of all human afflictions — cancer — would be next to fall. The overwhelming majority of Americans shared an unspoken assumption that twentieth-century medical science was on the verge of its greatest achievement yet: a cure for cancer. The cure would be perhaps a pill or an injection containing a chemical compound that could search out and destroy any cancerous tissue; or perhaps, as with polio, a preventive vaccine to immunize everyone against the disease. Maybe there would even be a chemically treated sugar cube to assure freedom from the fear and agony that cancer brings to hundreds of thousands of Americans each year.

We are a people who have become accustomed to the spectacular accomplishments of modern science: the discovery of penicillin in 1929; harnessing atomic power in 1945; overcoming polio in 1955; rocketing a man to the moon in 1969. It is not surprising that the common view, now decades old, is that a cure for cancer must certainly be within our grasp.

But the grim reality is otherwise. Despite the billions of dollars poured into cancer research in the United States and throughout the world, it is unlikely that there will be any sudden breakthrough in the near future. There will be no universal cure, no single vaccine against cancer. Certainly not in this decade. Probably not in this century. And possibly never.

Marked by tiny halting steps, progress in the search for a cancer cure is likely to follow a slow and uneven course. There will be little or no progress against some forms of the disease, perhaps slightly better results against other forms. Cancer, it seems, is not really a single disease susceptible to a single cure. It is a large group of separate diseases. It comes in many different forms, attacking scores of separate sites in the human body. True, all cancers do share a common characteristic — the uncontrolled growth of biologically destructive cells. And because of this common characteristic, there is always the chance that, unexpectedly, a scientist will stumble across a single agent that proves effective against all forms of the disease. That's the dream: a universal cure, a complete and final answer to the cancer enigma. But, realistically, the chances of that kind of miraculous discovery appear extremely remote. Certainly, public policy should not be founded on the anticipation of miracles. On the contrary, the most prudent public policy is to assume that despite the labor of the finest research scientists, the elusive universal cancer cure will remain beyond our grasp for the foreseeable future. Dr. Frank J. Rauscher, Jr., former Director of the National Cancer Institute, phrased it only slightly more optimistically in his 1974 report, when he told the Congress of the United States:

It is important to understand that research is not likely to produce a single dramatic means to prevent or cure all of the 100 or more forms of cancer.

Progress in science and medicine is a step-by-step process that takes time — time often measurable in years.

"Time often measurable in years." Unfortunately, the years have yielded little in the struggle against cancer. During the last twenty-five years of intensive pursuit of cancer cures, the survival rates for the most common types of cancer — lung cancer, breast cancer, and cancer of the colon — have remained almost unchanged. In the period 1950 to 1959, only 8 of every 100 victims of lung cancer survived for five years after diagnosis. In 1975, the five-year survival rate was only 9 out of 100. For the 89,000 women in 1975 who were told they have breast cancer, the five-year survival rate is expected to be 64 percent, a slight improvement over the 60 percent survival rate that existed two decades ago. With cancer of the colon — the most common of all major cancers, involving 100,000 new cases each year — the five-year survival rate was 44 percent between 1950 and 1959. Today, it is still about 44 percent.

In contrast with these dismal statistics, researchers point with justifiable pride to the improved survival rates for victims of leukemia and Hodgkin's disease. With the use of new drugs and experimental therapies, there has indeed been important progress in reducing the toll taken by these specific killers in recent years. But, regrettably, these life-saving victories are really at the distant edges of the overall battle against cancer, having far less impact than the public has been led to believe. As it turns out, Hodgkin's disease, a cancer of the lymphatic system, is one of the rarer forms of cancer. It accounts for just 1 percent of all cancer cases in the United States. As for leukemia, which accounts for 3 percent, or over 20,000 new cancer cases each year, the progress can be measured only with reference to the near hopelessness of the past. Current five-year survival rates are still tragically low: about 5 percent for acute leukemia and 30 percent for chronic leukemia.

What, then, is to be done? A great deal. There are two dimensions to the conquest of cancer. One dimension is to focus on a search for cures. That involves work largely in the realm of the unknown. The second dimension is to focus on the *causes* of cancer. Here, there is less mystery. In fact, our accumulated knowledge about the causes of cancer is very impressive, stretching back over 200 years. In 1775, a London physician, Percival Pott, first noted the apparent connection between exposure to coal soot among chimney sweeps and the subsequent high incidence of cancer of the scrotum among the young boys compelled to do this terrible work. Dr. Pott postulated that this malignancy, which was so common among chimney sweeps, must be attributable to the soot amassed on and within their bodies. The perceptive doctor was absolutely right, but it wasn't until this century that scientists isolated one of the cancer-causing chemicals present in coal soot — benzo(a)pyrene — the same substance that contaminates the air in many large cities and is deemed partially responsible for excessive rates of lung cancer among urban dwellers.

Coal soot and cancer: cause and effect. This was the first of the environmental cancer hazards to be identified. In 1822, another English physician, J. A. Paris, identified the connection between arsenic and skin cancer, a cause-and-effect relationship that is beyond dispute today. By the end of the nineteenth century, with the onrushing advance of the modern Industrial Age, scientists and physicians were just beginning to recognize the chemical origins of cancer: skin cancer among workers in the Scottish shale industry; cancer of the lip, larynx, and lung among workers handling coal tar and pitch; lung cancer, liver cancer, and bone cancer among miners of radioactive ore. In the 1930's, scientists singled out a number of chemical dyes as the cause of bladder cancer among dye workers. Shortly after that, during the 1940's and 1950's, with the accelerating pace of industrialization came a growing roster of demonstrated cancer-causing substances: many solvents, lubricants, and oil-based plastics; metals such as nickel and chromium; fibrous minerals such as asbestos; and radioactive substances. A collection of selected chemicals, metals, minerals and radioactive substances — these are the causative agents, the so-called carcinogens that act upon human cells, transforming them into ravenous, malignant entities, spreading and destroying life.

In the main, our heavy exposure to these carcinogens is directly related to the massive industrialization that has taken place with little regard for the health consequences to workers and the general public. Cancer is a disease as ancient as human history. But in the thousands of years of preindustrial life on earth, cancer hazards were relatively few, limited to a handful of natural carcinogens: the sun's ultraviolet radiation; radiation emanating from certain rocks; or naturally occurring arsenic that might be washed out of soil or rocks to contaminate food or water supplies. These natural cancer hazards still exist but they are dwarfed in significance by the new wave of carcinogens accompanying the industrialization and chemicalization of twentieth-century society. Cancer today, therefore, is actually a disease of man-made origin. What this means, of course, is that *cancer is largely a preventable disease.*

The man-made nature of the problem is underscored by National Cancer Institute estimates that the vast majority of all human cancers — perhaps up to 90 percent — are attributable to environmental carcinogens. If there is to be a twentieth-century breakthrough in the struggle against cancer, it will take the form of an early recognition that we must adopt national and state policies systematically limiting exposure to cancer-causing substances — at work, at home, and in the community. As things stand now, national public policy toward cancer fails to incorporate this mission of prevention. That is why it is a policy that is failing.

Cancer, once a relatively uncommon disease, now ranks second only to heart disease as the major cause of death in the United States. Last year over 370,000 Americans died of cancer and another 675,000 people were told for the first time that cancer had been discovered in their bodies. Each year both the death toll from cancer and the number of new cases are larger than the year before. These statistics reflect more than an increase of the American population or a greater proportion of old people within our population. Even after adjusting for these factors, the evidence is clear: cancer is on the rise, not only among the elderly but across all age categories — the middle-aged, young adults, and children.

For every twenty-five Americans who died in 1900, only one died of cancer. In 1975, nearly one of every five Americans who died was a victim of cancer. Unless we begin to make rapid headway in initiating preventive policies — in eliminating the known *environmental* causes of cancer — we can expect that of all Americans alive today at least one out of four, perhaps even one out of three, will die of cancer. In truth, what we are witnessing is the unmistakable emergence of a national cancer epidemic. An epidemic of frightful proportions. A cancer pox. The numbers and the trends point clearly to the calamity that is already upon us. But, of course, no statistical elaboration is adequate to convey the scope of this wrenching human tragedy. The victims themselves must be heard.

Contents

Part I

Chapter 1.

Joseph Fitman

A SIXTY-THREE-YEAR-OLD MAN should not have to work that hard, but there was really no choice. The company demanded it. The job demanded it. He put in six days a week, forty-eight hours, sometimes sixty hours a week. Once he worked seventy-two hours in a single week. A quiet man of good humor, Joseph Fitman was not a complainer. But he hated his job. He did the same dirty work all day long. He stood on a platform and sorted through large boxes of scrap rubber and plastic, looking for suitable pieces to set aside. Then he measured out an assortment of chemicals, pouring them from big heavy bags. When he had everything ready, he dumped it all into a huge machine called the bambury. Like a giant cement mixer, the bambury began to grind it all up. Amid dust and fumes and deafening noise, Joe Fitman then turned on a series of steam valves so that the scraps and chemicals would melt into a molten mass as they were grinding and mixing. He had to use enough steam to heat the mixture up to a temperature of more than 300 degrees. And while it was heating up he started over, as he had done thousands of times before, sorting and measuring for the next batch.

But this time would not be like the other times. While his eyes and fingers were searching through the boxes for more scraps, there was a muffled explosion, and the lid of the bambury suddenly flew open, spraying flaky pieces of hot rubber and plastic. Instinctively, Joe Fitman turned away, managing to shield his face, but, within seconds, he felt a searing pain on his right arm. When he looked, he saw little chunks of lavalike material burning into his skin. Quickly, he ran over to the foreman, who inspected the arm and told him to have it treated at a nearby community hospital and then go home.

During the short ride to the hospital the arm ached. And once in the hospital waiting room, the pain grew worse. He sat there for maybe an hour. Waiting. Pain. More waiting. When he finally got in to see the doctor, the examination was over almost as soon as it began. The medical treatment amounted to nothing more than washing the arm and wrapping it in gauze. On the way home the arm still hurt. But Joe Fitman figured he was pretty lucky. He knew it could have been a lot worse, especially if his face had been hit. And, anyway, today was Saturday, the sixth day, the last day, and he would be able to rest that evening and all day Sunday.

But there was no rest that Saturday night. His arm throbbed and ached and kept him from sleeping. By morning he felt rotten. The arm felt worse and he didn't feel like eating. Then that evening, he began to cough and couldn't stop. He coughed and coughed and grew sick to his stomach. Finally he threw up. He began coughing again and, this time, he spit up blood. He hated to tell his wife, Virginia, but he did. Then after another bad night — more coughing, more vomiting, and more blood — Virginia called the family doctor.

The doctor saw Joe Fitman the next day and immediately ordered a series of x-rays. By Friday, the doctor had carefully reviewed the results. He was clearly disturbed by what he saw and made arrangements for Joe Fitman to be admitted to Long Beach Memorial Hospital.

When he entered Long Beach Memorial, it was already eight days since the burn incident. By this time, Joe Fitman was weak. He hadn't been able to eat and he had lost nearly fifteen pounds. His symptoms suggested the possibility of tuberculosis, so he was confined to an isolation room. There, they began a seemingly endless stream of tests — x-rays, urine samples, blood tests, and then a bronchoscopy. The bronchoscopy was a miserable ordeal. The procedure required the patient to remain awake in a darkened room while the doctors slid a lighted tube over his tongue, down his throat, and into his lungs. The purpose of the bronchoscopy was to observe the interior of his lungs and take tissue samples. Despite a mild sedative to ease the discomfort, he could feel himself gagging and choking and on the verge of vomiting. Finally, after what seemed like an hour of probing, they removed the tube.

On his fifth day in the hospital, Joe Fitman learned he had lung cancer. Dr. Philip Wright, the surgeon assigned to the case, broke the news to him. The patient was calm but he had a number of questions. What would they do about the cancer? Surgery would be necessary. How far had the cancer gone? They wouldn't know until they operated. What were the chances? It was too early to tell, but the doctor was sure that at Joe's age he would have a rough road back. After hearing the answers to his questions, Joe Fitman voiced a common plea for a man in his situation. He told Dr. Wright to be sure to take out everything that looked cancerous. He didn't want any of it left to eat away at him.

There was to be another week of tests before the operation — blood tests, sputum samples, more urine tests — all to see if the cancer had spread to the liver, kidneys, or other vital organs.

The operation was performed on April 27, 1973. As it happened, that was Virginia Fitman's fifty-sixth birthday. Joe Fitman lay on the operating table face down as Dr. Wright cut into his left side until the upper part of his left lung was fully exposed. There, amid the maze of bronchial tubes reaching into the lung, the surgeon found a grayish mass: bronchogenic cancer. It was more than just a local tumor. The nearby lymph nodes in the bronchial tubes were enlarged and firm, apparently invaded by the spreading cancer. But there was still more. The cancer cells had reached up into the larynx, enveloping one of the vocal cords. Dr. Wright had little choice. He performed a radical left pneumonectomy — removal of the entire lung. In addition, he removed the cancerous vocal cord. The operation took nearly four hours.

For Joe Fitman, the next few days were a semiconscious blur. Most of the time he was oblivious to the activity around him. His wife was with him day and night. His children — six of them — took turns visiting. Nurses watched him closely, monitoring any changes. In several instances doctors were summoned to his bedside in the middle of the night. At times the physicians felt he wasn't going to make it; that his heart would simply stop under the strain of one lung trying to do the work of two.

Following the operation, Dr. Wright performed a tracheotomy, cutting a hole in the patient's throat and hooking up a respirator to do his breathing for him. Time and again, barely conscious, Joe Fitman would struggle to breathe on his own until his wife reminded him to relax and let the machine do it for him.

A week after his surgery, Joe Fitman was now alert enough to take some interest in himself and his condition. It was his weakness that most distressed him. Ten days after the operation, even though he was no longer dependent on a respirator, the smallest movement proved exhausting. Once he tried to slide off the bed and take two or three small steps to the bathroom. When he reached the toilet he was breathless and near collapse, having only enough strength left to reach up and press the emergency alarm button. A nurse ran to assist him, helped him back into bed, and then warned him not to even think about moving from bed without help.

Two and a half weeks after surgery, Joe Fitman went home. For days he lay in bed, unable to get up on his own. It wasn't until his third week at home that he had the strength to get to the bathroom unassisted. There, at last, he looked at himself in the mirror. He was appalled at what he saw. His skin was a grayish white. His medium-sized body, normally 170 pounds, had wasted away to 135 pounds. His skin looked lifeless, just hanging from his bones. He couldn't help but think that he looked more dead than alive.

Through that spring and summer of 1973, the recovery was slow and limited. But there were definite signs of improvement. He began to gain weight and with it some strength. He began to walk from one room to another, usually on his own. Occasionally, he would go outside to sit on the patio. Later, he and Virginia began to take walks down the block, stopping every few minutes so that he could get enough air to continue. It was slow, difficult, and frustrating, but Joe Fitman was getting better. His doctors were pleased with his progress, but it was clear he was never going to be the same. The cancer had required drastic surgery, and the quality of his life was permanently diminished by it.

Joe Fitman is sixty-five years old now. It has been almost two years since his lung cancer operation. Considering how gravely ill he was — and is — he looks surprisingly well. He is a lean man with dark hair that is graying and thinning. He wears thick glasses. He greets you with a firm handshake. But with a vocal cord gone, his voice is little more than a raspy whisper. And with only one weakened lung left to do the work of two, he has little energy for physical movement. When he coughs, the strain on his fragile respiratory system is evident. After nearly half a century as a laborer, Joseph Fitman is through. He'll never work again. Just managing to breathe and stay alive — survival — that's what his sixty-fifth year is all about.

He has a lot of time to think and talk now. Sitting. Thinking. Listening. Talking. These are the activities that fill up his days. If you ask him, he will tell you about his forty-nine years as an American worker. He tells the story slowly, deliberately. There are occasional pauses when his eyes take on a faraway look, while his mind reaches back over the years to recall the details. His is a story of a lifetime of hard work and pride. But at the end of it all, he received a cruel reward increasingly common among American workers: job-caused cancer.

As Joe Fitman begins to tell his story, you quickly forget about his raspy whisper. Instead, you hear his words and begin to see the picture they paint.

I quit school at the age of fifteen, against my dad's wishes. My mother had passed away before that. He wanted me to continue in school, but I wanted to go to work. After I did odd jobs with a friend of mine, I began work in an old-fashioned tin mill in Monessen, Pennsylvania. I worked in what's called the hot mill department, where they made sheets of tin. It must have been about 1926 when I started there. I was what they called a "single boy." My job was to grab the corner of the layered sheet iron with a pair of tongs — it was hot — and pull it off the roll to a place in front of another machine, the doubling machine. Then I would kick in the corner of the sheet to get the edge loose and I would pry up that hot tin to

*make sure the sheets wouldn't stick together. I was workin' with hot tin.
My work was hot. It wasn't heavy but it was sure hot, hot enough that I'd
go around with a cherry red nose and cherry red cheeks! I kind of liked
that work. It was hot, but I really liked that work.*

*I was there for years. But meanwhile, at Clairton, a town on the
Monongahela River, they was buildin' a huge automatic plant, a modern
strip mill, that would roll bars continuously into rolls of tin. Well, when
that plant was completed — I guess it was about 1936 — they went
ahead and opened up. Then they laid the plant off in Monessen, where I
lived. Anyway, they done away with the old-fashioned plants. At that
time, the Depression was already on, and everything in that town was
slacked down, and I found myself unemployed. Virginia and I had only
been married a few months. I couldn't get work, so I was forced on relief.*

*Then Roosevelt come out with this WPA, and I managed to get on the
WPA. I worked there about two or three years. I was a laborer. I worked
on a road — construction on a road. Then I worked in a stone quarry for
the WPA. It was heavy work, pryin' out huge stones with a bar. It was
like you see in a prison, men breakin' stone, workin' on the rockpile! They
broke that stone up for use in roads, and we'd shovel it in a truck, and the
truck would take it out. Sometimes in winter there'd be snow all around.
You'd have no feelin' in your toes. They'd have to send us home. The
WPA was only payin' me sixty-two dollars a month, but it was better than
bein' unemployed. We all lived pretty good when we were on WPA. At
least we had food on the table and we had gas in our car.*

*Well, anyway, while I was with the WPA I had an application in with
the American Chain and Cable Company. They called me up. As a matter of fact, there was a knock on the door one evening. There was a man
at the door, a security guard. He gave me a paper and said, "You can
start to work tomorrow." It was very lucky, too, because our first daughter
was born that August, 1940.*

*I worked as a laborer at American Chain and Cable for about a year
before they sent me up to the blacksmith's shop. I worked as a blacksmith's
helper. I tried to be such a good helper, and it got me to be a blacksmith.
The blacksmith . . . Marsden . . . that was his name, he was in his late
sixties at that time. At first he was — well, he was cranky. Nothin' pleased
him. He was hard to get along with. But after a while he took a likin' to
me. I reminded him of his son-in-law.*

He was very bright. He was a wonderful handsome man . . . gray hair like what you see in the ads in the paper . . . suits advertised for older men. He taught me everything. Actually, he didn't exactly teach me. I myself learned the trade by watchin' him. I kept my eyes open. Many times I'd go home and pick a pencil up and start figurin' out how he'd know how to cut exactly the right amount off the billet to make a forgin'.

He was a wise man. But he had the habit of — mostly on weekends — goin' out on a drunk, goin' to different clubs drinkin' to the point where he'd come to work Monday mornin's in his bedroom slippers! He'd tell me, "Joe, you know what to do." Then he'd go right between the furnace and the wall where it was covered and all warm and he'd go to sleep there. And eventually, later on, he would wake up and come out of there smackin' his lips 'cause of the bad taste in his mouth!

Anyway, when he left I stepped in and took over. I worked there for just about sixteen years, from 1940 to 1956. When the war was on they would've drafted me right away, but I was deferred on account of my job. I was needed as a blacksmith — forgin' material, temperin' material. I was needed. A blacksmith's work — you've got to be more intelligent than some. There's a lot of mathematics involved. While I was at work, I attended night school. It was a credentialed school, and I took up drafting — mechanical drafting — while I was at work. Thus, when I went to work in the blacksmith's shop, I already had education in layout and mathematics. In other words, I could figure out how to cut a four-inch square billet. I just know how much to cut off of that piece of steel to make that forgin'. I'd do it on paper plus in my head . . .

I also forged huge cutting tools for the roll shop. I had to forge it to the right dimension. Then I had to temper that cutting tool. I was important. I loved that work. It reminds me of a story Marsden told me. One day, this was in Scotland, the king wanted to find out who was the most important man in Scotland. So he called all the important people together, and each one took their turn tryin' to persuade him. First a big butcher kneeled in front of the king holdin' a huge cleaver in one hand and sayin', "With this cleaver I butcher the meat you eat. Without me you would go hungry." Then a carpenter come before him holdin' a hammer and nails and says, "Without me you wouldn't have a castle to live in." Then a doctor comes up to the king pointin' to his scissors and other fine steel instruments and he says, "Without me you wouldn't get the surgery

*you need to keep you healthy." Finally, here comes up an old man, a
gray-haired blacksmith wearin' a leather apron. He bows before the king
and says, "Your Majesty, these people have all had their say-so, but without me where would they all be? I made the butcher's cleaver. I made the
carpenter's tools. And I made the doctor's instruments. Without me these
fellas would be helpless. They wouldn't have the tools they need to do their
work." And right there the king proclaimed the blacksmith the most important man in Scotland!*

*I loved that work. Well, anyway, I was a good steady worker. I didn't
drink, and for sixteen years I always showed up on my job. But then something developed in my work. One of my helpers refused to cooperate with
me and made trouble for me at my work and kept me back from doin' the
work I was supposed to do, which upset me. And I couldn't come to terms
with the company foreman and the head of the union — I was a union
member. I was a union member, but they didn't help in the dispute I had
. . . It would take too long to explain, but I was upset.*

When his mother-in-law offered financial help if they moved
to California, Joe was ready. At the time they sold their house
and left Monessen, the Fitmans were a family of seven, Joe and
Virginia and five children. Crowded into a 1954 Mercury and
pulling a trailer full of belongings, they drove to Long Beach,
California, where they quickly settled down.

The Long Beach area is part of the vast industrial, commercial, and residential underbelly of Los Angeles County. It is part
of a sprawling fifteen-mile east-west collection of oil refineries,
shipyards, aircraft companies, and thousands of miscellaneous
manufacturing plants — all of it interspersed with the modest
homes and apartments that shelter a work force numbering into
the hundreds of thousands.

Within a few weeks of their arrival in California, the Fitmans
bought a house. The price was $15,600: $2600 down and $84 a
month. The house itself was part of a large tract of homes, a
comfortable stucco structure complete with a two-car garage.
After their children had all grown, Joe and Virginia still lived in
that same house on Poppy Street in Long Beach.

At the time, the move west in 1956 seemed to be a leg up on

the good life. Less than two decades before, Joe had worked for the WPA for $62 a month. Yet, here they were, a family of seven moving into a four-bedroom house located less than ten miles from the Pacific Ocean beaches.

But the job situation was not as cheery. In Monessen, Joe had job security and a job he loved. In California, he was increasingly plagued by two new realities over which he had absolutely no control: layoffs and his own advancing age.

We moved into this house when we came out here. We had five-and-a-half children — Virginia was about six months pregnant when we came out here. But we were all happy to come out . . . Well, after about a month or two I wrote to the union that this seemed to be a healthy place for the family as well as for myself. And I wrote also to the company back east that I decided to stay here. I got a wonderful letter from the company as well as the union. The letter I got from the company . . . I could show that to any industry . . . and, well, I was proud of that letter for what they thought of me back there. I don't know what I done with that letter. To this day, I don't know what ever happened to it. I guess I don't need it now.

But, anyway, comin' out here in 1956 I got a job workin' for Reisner Forge Company. They're up here in South Gate, just about seven miles from me. We were here for only a week when I got the job at the employment agency. I went in and I worked there as a steam-hammer driver and they didn't ask me if I was a blacksmith. I was laid off there in 1957 with two other fellas due to a work shortage. But when I was laid off, my supervisor — the head of the shop — told me they had to lay me off due to seniority. He told me to keep close tabs with him. . .

After leavin' that place up there, I was out of work for seven months. Meanwhile, I was gettin' older. I was close to fifty. Finally, I was hired to work for Douglas Aircraft. When I was hired, I learned how to work on a bench saw. One thing about Douglas — it was close enough so that I could ride a bike to work. I loved that. I actually got a big kick out of ridin' a bicycle. Matter of fact, when John Kennedy was runnin' for President in 1960, I was ridin' my bicycle on Lakewood through the crowds when he was speakin' there. I liked Kennedy. I've been a Democrat but believe it or not I haven't voted since I came out here. I look at it now, since this Watergate goin' on and all — it's sickening what's goin' on in this country. If you're a real patriot — American — when you used to sit at dinner places and hear "God Bless America" — sometimes it almost makes tears come to your eyes.

Anyway, I worked there at Douglas Aircraft for a little better than three years. I operated a saw, cuttin' fiber glass. It was a pretty good job but it was on the dirty side. We weren't ordered to wear a mask but we were ordered to wear a shield or glasses due to the material comin' at you off of the saw. So you see, I could have been breathin' some of that. That was a union job, under the Auto Workers. After so many weeks, you became a member of the union. The wages weren't bad. I started out at $2.56 and went up to $2.68.

I got along well with the fellas there. I was well liked. One day at Douglas we were out eatin' our lunch and, jokingly, I said to the guys, "I wonder if Douglas is goin' to shut down tomorrow." They said, "Why?" and I said, "'Cause it's my birthday." The very next day we were eatin' our lunch again, and they gave me this beautifully wrapped box with a birthday card on it. When I opened the box, it was a beautiful shirt inside. Those fellas had taken up a collection and went out and bought that shirt for me.

Well, I worked there at Douglas for three years. Then after three years they begin to catch up with all of their orders, such as those big orders, orders for a hundred-and-some DC-8's. They were catchin' up with them orders. Things began to slack up. They didn't need all their workers which ran well over 20,000 that were employed at Douglas. Well, they begin to have layoffs every week on Fridays. They would lay off 900 men and then the following week 1200. Every week you were worried it would be you. Finally, it come to where they caught up to me. I still had faith that I'd make it because I was older in seniority than the two other men who worked with me. I figured they'd have to be let go first, and, by then, they might get some orders in before they catch up to me. Well, when next week come they didn't lay off only them two other guys. They got all three of us!

Joe was unemployed for most of 1961. He was fifty-two years old and desperate for work. After seven months of looking, he finally got a job. It was his last job and his worst. The outfit that hired him was Collins, Caldwell & Dague, a small company involved in specialized reclamation. Collins, Caldwell & Dague bought thousands of pounds of rubber and vinyl scraps — defective water beds, broken phonograph records, galoshes, chunks of broken plastic. They melted these materials and reconstituted them for use by manufacturing firms that require vast quantities of plastics. Toy manufacturers and firms making phonograph records were big purchasers.

Joe Fitman's job was to operate the bambury machine. The work was dirty, exhausting, and ultimately dangerous.

One thing about that place, it was always dusty and dirty. It's a shame how filthy. Well, I'd be dirty immediately. Some of the guys used to take showers before they'd go home and they were dirty again before they got home. The dirt would come out from all the chemicals that was delivered there in a cart and put in the corners — stashed away. They were all ready for use in fiber drums, boxes, and bags — fifty-pound bags and twenty-five-pound bags. They had this carbon black in fifty-pound bags, and there was some that also come in twenty-five-pound bags. The twenty-five-pound bags was the powdery form. It was like a woman's powder. And that was nasty because you would pour it, and the dust would come up in your face.

I had a bow knife and while I went ahead and put the vinyl scrap material in the machine, I would get a bag of carbon black and cut it across and shake the contents into the bambury while it was operating. And I'd get another bag of whatever it called for, cut it, and empty it. Then I would put the lever down — put pressure on the material inside the bambury. With the steam heat and with it grindin', why it would bring it up to mush material, big bulk. I had a gauge up there — that's my heat and temperature gauge. It had on there degrees — from zero to 400 degrees. Well, now, that's where your experience is. When you experience what different type of material you're goin' to work with, it would indicate when it was ready to be dropped on the conveyor belt for the rest of the workingmen down below.

It was continuous work. While one load was cookin' — it takes about ten minutes for that to cook — it took me just about ten minutes to pull apart the scrap. It had to be cleaned. There was some adhesive tape which

I'd throw aside. Glasses, bottles, soda pop, empty cans — I had to sort that out. And I'd have another bag of material ready while I'm doin' this sortin'. Sometimes I had a scale which required eighteen pounds of this white lead or something like that. I'd get that ready. Meanwhile, the material already in the bambury is cookin' and it's ready to drop. Sometimes I got to hurry up to keep track because I've got to have it ready to dump in. And I'm doin' this all day.

At break time, the other fellas would share. One fella would take care of things while the other fella went out to the side of the plant where they would have a catering truck and would help theirselves eat. But I couldn't. I was the only one that worked through steady. I had too much to do. I've got to measure this stuff like I told you. I had to hurry up 'cause they couldn't afford it to stop. It was continuous. I was faced with that and I had been doin' that until the point where I got . . .

There were no breaks. I'd try to eat lunch in between batches of material. I'd hurry up to eat and keep my eye . . . make sure I already had the material cooked and shut off, ready to drop when they're ready. I always made sure I already had another batch ready. And only then could I eat. I'd unwrap my sandwich up on the platform, take two bites, wrap it up, put it aside, keep workin', weighin' material. How would you like to dip a coffee can into a bag, weigh the material on the scale and set that can down, brush your hands on your clothes which are all dirty, open the sandwich and eat it and see black fingerprints on the white bread? I had to put up with that. Virginia doesn't know the several times I just threw it away. I wasn't eatin' right.

Anyway, these young fellas, I've seem them come and go. They didn't put up with that. When a young fella would come in lookin' for work, I would confront him and say, "What the hell is a young fella like you doin' in here?" And they asked me, "How do you like it here?" I'd shake my head, "If I was twenty years younger I wouldn't be in here." I told them young fellas straight. Now there was some fellas stuck it out for several months. But then they disappeared, gave up.

Well, I handled that carbon black . . . and all kinds of things up there on the platform. I would just pour it down into the bambury. My plant had no air conditioner or ventilation system. The only thing they had was a tin roof. They had sky vents, about four in that plant. But they kept that closed all the time because they didn't want none of that material to go out. *It would blow out and the people in that area would complain, 'cause they did one time. There'd be so much dust sometimes the office workers at my company would have black around their eyes — looked like raccoons! One time, on these dusty conditions, my foreman . . . told me they were complainin' about that dust in the office. He come up to me. He says, "Joe, is there any way of cuttin' that out?" I said, "Well, that little suction innovation," and I leaned over the bambury, "it can't take care of all that. All of that steam and dust comin' out . . ." I told him, "The best thing would be to build a big hood, a tin hood over my head and have a fan up there to draw that up." But they couldn't see it. They just said no.*

The only thing I could do is bear with it. I tried their masks. They — I couldn't — my glasses steamed up. I tried a rag tied around. From my point of view, that place is filthy up there. And I just wonder, throughout this country, if the rest of the places are like that. You can't complain 'cause you got to watch your job. If you did complain they would get rid of you. A fella's got to watch his mouth, you know. Otherwise he's out. No union protection. I don't know who's the head of the health operation in the United States, but they should look into it, should make rules for the guys that are workin' there, get off their butts and see that something's done about the health hazards. About the only guy that ever came around was a fire inspector.

I begin to cough a lot while I was at work, gradually to cough more and more about nine or ten years ago. Black. Always black. Virginia would give me the devil if I didn't wash my spit down the sink. I thought I washed it down. But that black would be awful. I tried, but your body can't throw things like that aside when you're up in age.

I don't know what was the ingredients in the material we ran. Only a chemist that made the formula . . . he could have added . . . anything to that material. We didn't know. I didn't know what the material was made up of — except we had to keep movin' to put out production. In a way I knew the materials I was workin' with was dangerous, but when you're up in age like me . . .

There was a few others there, but we had to make a livin'. We also knew that if we lost our job there it'd be hard to find work elsewhere on account of our age. I had no other means of support for my family due to my age and havin' no skill. Just a tradesman. They didn't have blacksmiths out here.

I was told by a doctor eight to ten years ago — he looked at my x-rays and told me that I had black lungs. He ordered me off of cigarettes. He told me that if it's possible to get the hell off of that job. But like I said, despite all things, keep goin'. Your age is against you. You've got a house payment. You've got six kids around the table. You've got to have an income. And the only way you get an income is work for it.

In the months after his operation — during the spring and summer of 1973 — as Joe Fitman's prospects for survival improved, he was a man beset by worries. There was his physical condition — weakness, difficulty in breathing — and concealed fears about whether the cancer might recur. There was also the matter of the family's finances. The medical and hospital bills were only partially covered by insurance. This left a personal debt of more than $2000. And the bills were still piling up. State disability benefits amounted to $105 per week. But after six months, those benefits ran out. There was a pending workmen's compensation claim, but that had been bogged down for months. So, at sixty-four years of age, still one year short of his full social security and Medicare benefits, Joe Fitman decided to file for unemployment. But that meant he had to look for work again.

After my surgery, when I was no longer eligible for disability, I had to turn to unemployment. I followed the rules. I looked for work. But them places would take one look at me and say, "Forget it." They looked at me like I was an old nag showin' up for the Kentucky Derby!

When I started drawin' unemployment, the state people — they interviewed me and they asked me if I can do this and that. And I said, "It has to be light work. I could look for work and do light work, such as security guard or something where I wouldn't have to be rushin' or pick up over twenty-five pounds." Well, when I told her this, the woman interviewin' me said, "Just a moment." She called up a place that hires security guards and she said, "I have a man here" — she described my injury. They say no, no. They can't use me. They're not hirin'. Then she said to me, "Just a moment." She called up where I worked, where all this took place, and she said, "Let me talk to the assistant supervisor." Jack was his

*name. He talked to her, and she asked, "Jack, do you have something
light for Joe?" And he told her down there, "No. All we have is heavy
work." They wouldn't take me back. In other words, like a horse, if he's
washed up he goes to the glue factory!*

*Anyway, that's it. We're not treated as humans. The majority of us in
this country, we're only good as long as we can do our work. And if we
stumble, they push us aside and put a younger part in there. A younger
machine. So we're actually like machines. We got to keep goin'. When
we're wore out they get a new one for you.*

For many months, the financial drain continued without
letup. Finally, halfway into 1974 — fourteen months after the
surgery — there was a happy turn of events. In the case of
Joseph Fitman v. *McDonnell-Douglas Corporation; Collins, Caldwell & Dague/Kamco;* et al, the California Workmen's Compensation Appeals Board approved a compensation settle-
ment. On June 17, 1974, Joseph Fitman received a lump-sum
award of $23,332.82. That same day he turned sixty-five, enti-
tling him to both social security retirement benefits and the all
important Medicare coverage. Joseph Fitman, his body broken
and worn out, had made it to senior citizenship — what retirement hucksters used to call "the golden years."

What of his life at this time?

*I can't do too much. Mostly, I just watch TV or walk to the patio — sit
down. Or Virginia and I both get in the car and go somewhere. I tried to
work, but I just can't 'cause I'm fightin' so many things. If I do too much,
I wind up goin' to the hospital in an emergency. I get the feelin' like if you
ran around this block, stopped, sat down, you'd be takin' deep breaths.
Well, that's my problem. I get spells where my air was bein' shut off and I
feel I'm not gettin' oxygen, and I found myself strugglin' for some air.
Well, that's the sensation I have, havin' one lung.*

*But right now everything seems to be all right. In a way I'm enjoyin'
retirement. I'm not sorry I retired from that job. But I feel sorry for the
fellas that are tryin' to hold their jobs in that area because only I know,
due to my experience, how dangerous that place is to work.*

So right now my future is . . . I'm just retired. I'm past sixty-five now and I'm up in age. I can't do no work. My age is against me. My health is against me. The only thing I could do is show a fella, like in my line of work, show a fella how to do it . . . the blacksmith's work. You see, I was an important man there. I already told you the story about the blacksmith in Scotland — the most important man. Well, I feel the same way. My work was important — and it was important because in the 1940's when the Second World War broke out, they took in doctors. Medical doctors. Machinists. Electricians. They were all drafted. Lawyers. They all were drafted. But I got a card there . . . deferred on account of my work. It was essential. I was needed for the war, to keep the supplies goin' out.

My work was interesting. I could make so many things, like tools and star drills. I think back often. I loved that work. I think back on some of the . . . actually you will too. You'll think back to this. You'll think back to — you probably forgot — the most important man in Scotland.

Well, it's been a good life.

Chapter 2.

Job-Caused Cancer

ON THE EVENING OF MARCH 30, 1975, after a month in the hospital, Joe Fitman died. Tests and radiation treatments had proved a vain effort to cope with the recurrence of respiratory cancer. He had been good about it all, complaining only of a continuing pain in his chest, something different from the usual shortness of breath he had experienced for so many months. After his death, a pathologist performed an autopsy that revealed what had been happening inside Joe's body. The cancer that was once confined to the larynx and bronchial area had spread to his heart, choking off his arteries. Choking off their ability to carry blood from his heart. Choking off what little life remained.

Three days later, family and friends, perhaps seventy-five people, attended funeral services for Joe Fitman. He lay in an open casket, dressed in a dark suit, remarkably handsome in death. The pastor spoke of an end to the hospitals and the pain and suffering. In his words, "Brother Joe is now at the gateway to a better place." And then the fitting lyrics from the Christian gospel:

> Precious Lord, take my hand,
> Lead me on, help me stand;
> I am tired, I am weak, I am worn;
> Thru the storm, thru the night,
> Lead me on to the light;
> Take my hand, precious Lord, lead me home.

Soon after, the casket was sealed and taken to the graveside. A few more words were spoken to the tearful gathering. The flowers atop the casket were wrapped in white ribbons. On one ribbon was written "Beloved Husband." On another "Beloved Father."

It was all over for Joe Fitman. But his story must not stop here. The hospital records, the autopsy report, the death certificate — on the surface their cryptic notations suggest a routine case of a man who simply grew sick and died. But there is more to it than that. A close analysis of the record — a searching review of Joe Fitman's work history — reveals that the cancer that ultimately took his life was not simply an isolated misfortune. Quite the contrary. The cancer that killed this man was almost certainly directly related to the jobs he held and the work he did during forty-nine years of industrial labor.

Joe Fitman could not have known it at the time, but when he toiled for a quarter-century as a hot metal worker, first as a teen-ager in a Pennsylvania tin mill and later as a blacksmith in a steel mill, he was working in a high-risk occupational cancer environment. Long-time metal workers, their lungs assaulted by iron oxides and a host of metallic dusts and fumes, develop lung cancer at rates significantly higher than the general population. In 1962, the University of Pittsburgh undertook a massive study to investigate the relationship between the causes of death among steelworkers and their work histories. The study systematically followed a population of 58,828 men who had been employed in seven steel plants in 1953. By 1962, a distinct pattern was evident. The study revealed that cancer of the lungs, bronchus, and trachea was killing white steelworkers at a rate 28 percent greater than in the general population. For nonwhite workers — those generally relegated to the dirtiest jobs — the rate was 64 percent greater than in the general population. Some workplaces proved to be far more dangerous than others, so-called hot spots for cancer. The work area where Joe Fitman labored for sixteen years — the blacksmith's shop — produced cancer of the lung, bronchus, and trachea at a rate two-and-a-half times what would normally be expected. What does this mean in human terms? Instead of finding the "expected" number of these cancer cases — 3 for every 100 deaths — nearly 8 out of 100 were dying from these cancers. In the cold terminology of the biostatisticians, the blacksmith's shop was the source of a startling number of "excess" cancer deaths.

Joe Fitman could not have known that. Nor could he have known the hazards he faced when, in 1958, he took the job as a bench saw operator with Douglas Aircraft in Long Beach.

We weren't ordered to wear a mask but we were ordered to wear a shield or glasses due to the material comin' at you off of the saw. So you see, I could have been breathin' some of that.

He was indeed "breathin' some of that." He was inhaling millions of tiny fiber-glass particles in the course of a work day, the fiberglass particles that are now suspect as a cancer-causing agent.

Finally, in 1961, after he had been laid off at Douglas, Joe took his last job — operating the bambury machine at Collins, Caldwell & Dague. There, daily, for twelve years, he had to handle or breathe a variety of toxic agents, including gases emanating from melting plastics and carbon black, a commercially produced sootlike substance widely used to reinforce rubber. Joe called carbon black "nasty" because "it was like a woman's powder . . . you would pour it, and the dust would come up in your face." He did not know that carbon black is also a suspect carcinogen.

Which of these multiple exposures, spanning tens of thousands of working hours, was chiefly responsible for the cancer that killed Joe? We can never know for sure. Cancer is not like a car accident or the collapse of a bridge. There are no eyewitnesses to the destructive impact of a carcinogen upon the tissue in someone's lung. But this much we do know: rarely, if ever, is cancer a spontaneous disaster. Instead, virtually every cancer is the product of repeated and cumulative carcinogenic insults to individual human cells. Joe Fitman's work history provided a steady succession of these carcinogenic insults.

The cancerization process is as subtle as it is insidious. Hidden from view, the process of biologic violence begins with cells under siege. Cells. The human body is made up of billions of cells, tiny microscopic units of life that take carbohydrate fuel — oxygen-bearing sugar — and transform it into the indispensable energy that enables a heart to beat, a lung to breathe, and a brain to think. In her environmental classic, *Silent Spring,* the late biologist Rachel Carson observed that each human cell can be likened to "a chemical factory which is one of the wonders of the living world." How is it that in Joe Fitman's body some normal cells — those wondrous "chemical factories" — went awry, triggering a deadly journey ending in an uncontrollable malignant tumor?

For Joe Fitman the cancerization process may have begun as long ago as forty-five years before his death. It was then, when he was not yet twenty years old, that his body was subjected to daily doses of carcinogens common to certain types of hot metal work. We now know that the site of a cancer is largely dependent upon the nature of the carcinogen involved and its route of exposure. Some carcinogens are most reactive with the cells of the skin; for example, arsenic has long been known to cause skin cancer. Other carcinogens, most notably the so-called aromatic amines used in dyestuff and rubber operations, are highly reactive in the urinary bladder, ultimately leading to bladder cancer. Still other carcinogens assault the blood-and-lymph-forming tissues, causing leukemia, lymphoma, or Hodgkin's disease. As it happened, Joe Fitman's principal exposure was in breathing a series of airborne carcinogens that are most reactive with the tissue in the respiratory system. These carcinogens were silently, relentlessly bombarding the cells in his bronchial tubes, beginning a process that slowly but irreversibly altered their essential structure. The cells now bore a carcinogenic imprint that, in turn, they transmitted to each succeeding generation of cells. Over the years, the normal cells gave way to generations of abnormal cells and, finally, to a generation of cancerous cells: cells targeted and programmed to wreak biologic havoc. Cancerization. Cells, which were once the building blocks of life, giving rise to cells that have become the opposite of life. Their growth and appetite are uncontrolled. They clump together in tumors. They spread in crablike fashion, invading adjacent tissue. And then, unchecked, they metastasize; that is, some of these malignant cells may break away to be carried in the bloodstream and lymph channels, reaching distant organs where they lodge and grow and spread further. In the end, cancerization means the cell has become the anticell. Life has become antilife. And, finally, the body succumbs to the invasion. Death.

This, then, is the general outline of the cancerization process. Of course, not everyone who sustains prolonged exposure to one or more carcinogens contracts cancer. Some individuals appear to be more "cancer-resistant" than others, just as some of us manage to ward off colds and viruses better than others. If it had been simply a matter of Joe Fitman's exposure to carcinogens as a metal worker, he might have never been struck by cancer. Those exposures alone may not have been sufficient to cause the disease. But the years of hot metal work were followed by the fiber-glass exposure at Douglas, and then the very heavy contact with a series of chemicals at Collins, Caldwell & Dague. With at least half a dozen carcinogens implicated in this particular case, it is virtually impossible to sort out the role played by each of these separate cancer-causing agents. Nevertheless, the history here points to an inescapable conclusion: The total carcinogenic burden — that is, the decades of cumulative biologic insults inflicted by these workplace carcinogens — was too great for Joe Fitman's body to withstand. The result: cells gone mad. A killer cancer.

In 1942, a little-known German-born pathologist, Dr. Wilhelm C. Hueper, wrote a monumental 896 page text entitled *Occupational Tumors and Allied Diseases.* Drawing upon hundreds of animal studies and studies of selected worker populations, Hueper convincingly established the relationship between occupational contact with certain chemicals, metals, and minerals and the subsequent high incidence of cancer among exposed workers. In recalling the nature of his research, Hueper later observed that he spent years poring over every available study, both here and abroad. As he put it, "one piece of dirt led to another" until, finally, after four years of research, he felt justified in publishing a comprehensive categorization of the principal cancer-causing substances threatening industrial workers.

A tireless public health advocate, Hueper did not stop there. His book was more than a scientific tome; in its pages he pleaded for action, urging the adoption of strict preventive measures to minimize the cancer hazards faced by working men and women. Regrettably, his advocacy had little effect.

During the late 1940's and throughout the 1950's, the evidence mounted in support of Hueper's theory on the origins of cancer. Still, despite the persuasive body of evidence, for the most part public health authorities remained unmoved. By this time, Hueper had himself become Chief of the National Cancer Institute's Environmental Cancer Section and an embattled pioneer in the field of occupational cancer. In 1964, at the age of seventy, he coauthored a second massive text, this one entitled *Chemical Carcinogenesis and Cancers.* In it, Hueper wrote ominously of an impending "epidemic in slow motion." He noted, emphasized, and then reemphasized the fact that human cancer ordinarily does not appear until ten, twenty, or even thirty or forty years after exposure to a carcinogen. Because of this extraordinarily long latent period, he warned that unless immediate and effective controls were applied, the unbridled proliferation of cancer-causing substances, which accompanied the frenetic industrialization in the years since 1940, would, in time, produce a terrible cancer epidemic in the United States. It now appears that a continuing policy of national neglect, joined with the passage of time, is proving Hueper right. Consider for a moment this partial registry of human loss:

• Rubber workers, routinely exposed to multiple cancer-causing substances, are dying of cancer of the stomach, cancer of the prostate, and leukemia and other cancers of the blood-and-lymph-forming tissues at rates ranging from 50 percent to 300 percent greater than in the general population.

• Steelworkers, particularly the thousands who handle coal as it is transferred to coke ovens for combustion and distillation, fall victim to kidney and lung cancer at excessive rates. Those who labor atop the hot coke ovens are most vulnerable to the carcinogenic coal tar emissions. Instead of dying from lung cancer at the expected rate of 3 or 4 out of 100, at least 20 out of every 100 die from the disease.

• Asbestos workers, including those who mill this mineral fiber and those who must use it regularly in construction work and elsewhere, die from lung cancer at a rate more than seven times that of comparable control groups. Mesothelioma, a fatal malignancy that attacks the lining of the lungs and abdominal organs, used to be an extremely rare form of cancer. But now it has become a relatively commonplace cause of death for asbestos workers, even among those with short-term occupational exposures.

• Workers who produce dyestuffs, using benzidine and other related chemicals, have evidenced notoriously high rates of urinary bladder cancer. In a study of a group of dyestuff workers who were exposed to benzidine and beta-Naphthylamine for five years or more, nearly all of them — 94 percent — later developed bladder tumors.

• The picture is nearly as depressing among certain groups of miners. Miners of uranium, iron ore, nickel, chromium, and other industrial metals succumb to a wide range of occupationally induced cancers. In the case of uranium miners, the lung cancer rate is astonishing, accounting for upwards of 50 percent of all deaths.

• An estimated two million workers, among them dry cleaners, painters, printers, rubber and petroleum workers, are exposed to the solvent benzene, a known leukemia-producing agent. Another 1.5 million laborers, among them insecticide workers, farmworkers, and copper and lead smelter workers, are exposed to inorganic arsenic, a carcinogen that causes high rates of lung, skin and lymphatic cancer. In addition, machinists, chemical workers, woodworkers, roofers — and many, many more — join an ever-expanding list of workers who hold jobs posing special cancer risks of one kind or another.

Predictably, cancer trends tend to appear first among blue-collar workers because they are usually the first to encounter intense and prolonged exposure to both the older and the newer cancer-causing substances. And so it is that while the national cancer epidemic is just recently an emerging phenomenon, among blue-collar workers the epidemic has long since passed beyond its incipient stages. Workers — miners, agricultural workers, industrial workers — when they enter the workforce they are among the strongest and healthiest of citizens. They are the ones who should ordinarily be living into their seventies and eighties, even into their nineties. But instead they fall victim to occupational disease — often occupational cancer — and by the tens of thousands, die in their sixties or fifties and sometimes in their forties or thirties. Victims of blue-collar cancer.

Where were the guardians of the public's health while this epidemic of blue-collar cancer was in the making? For decades federal and state health agencies treated occupational cancer as a nonissue or, at best, a relatively inconsequential side-issue. To some extent, this conduct can be attributed to the fact that, like the general public, many health officials were lulled into believing that a universal cancer cure was in the offing, some kind of dramatic knockout punch that would obviate the need for costly preventive policies. But a more telling explanation rests with the tendency of key public officials to act in tandem with industry's spokesmen. In a twisted notion of the public interest, they consciously endeavor to play down the specter of occupational cancer, lest it "frighten" workers and possibly impair production.

In this regard, Dr. Hueper's own experiences are highly instructive. In 1948, six years after the publication of his work, *Occupational Tumors and Allied Diseases,* Dr. Hueper was appointed Chief of the Environmental Cancer Section of the National Cancer Institute. Amid the then burgeoning enthusiasm surrounding atomic power, Hueper harbored the gravest concerns about the evidence of severe lung cancer hazards to uranium workers. One of his first efforts at the National Cancer Institute was to initiate a proposed investigation of cancer rates among uranium ore miners in the Rocky Mountains. With the study well underway, the doctor was invited to present a paper to a meeting of the Colorado State Medical Society. The subject: environmental and occupational cancer hazards on the Colorado Plateau. In his draft, Hueper referred to the European studies dating back to 1879, which indicated almost unbelievable lung cancer rates among radioactive ore miners, attack rates ranging from 40 to 75 percent of exposed miners. Because of objections from the Atomic Energy Commission, administrators at the National Cancer Institute ordered Dr. Hueper to delete any mention of these studies. In the Atomic Energy Commission's view, dissemination of such information among members of the Colorado medical profession was not in the public interest. Finding these developments irreconcilable with his conscience as a scientist, Dr. Hueper withdrew from the speaking engagement rather than deliver a censored speech.

Another far more serious incident occurred in 1952. It apparently grew out of Dr. Hueper's prior studies that demonstrated rampant lung cancer among American chromate workers. Hueper and others eventually found the lung cancer incidence among white workers employed in one large chromate-producing plant to be forty times normal; among nonwhite workers the lung cancer rate was eighty times normal. This finding served as one further piece of evidence implicating the entire chromate industry in what appeared to be a major outbreak of occupational cancer. It is a long way from the mining of chromate ore to the shiny chrome plating on a new automobile. Hueper knew that in this chain of industrial operations — and in scores of other industrial operations involving chromate and chromium compounds — tens of thousands of workers become potential cancer victims. Chromium. Uranium. It seemed to Hueper that the dimensions of the entire occupational cancer problem were mushrooming before his eyes. Evidently, the meaning of his research was not lost on those whose economic interests he threatened. Dr. Hueper recalls what happened:

> My active direction of epidemiologic studies on occupational cancer hazards and cancers in American industries was forcefully and abruptly brought to a halt in 1952 by an order of the Surgeon General . . . [This followed] a protest to the Public Health Service by the medical advisor to the chromate-producing industry, on behalf of his clients. In this protest, promoted by the industry as an action of "self defense," it was alleged that my activities were detrimental to their interests. As the result of this intervention by a medical consultant of private industry, I

was forbidden to contact thereafter state health departments and industrial concerns on all matters of occupational cancer. [I was ordered] to discontinue all field work on this subject and to restrict my activities entirely to experimental research . . . in the laboratory.

This order, relegating Hueper to work far removed from the front lines of any assault on occupational cancer, was never rescinded. It stood as an example of the ease with which private industry could persuade public officials to limit the possible impact of a scientist's work. In a 1959 speech, prepared for delivery to the Executive Council of the AFL-CIO, a determined Dr. Hueper — still the embattled Chief of the Environmental Cancer Section — described the disastrous effect of these events on the effort to identify the occupational origins of many cancers.

The cold fact is that since 1952 the successor organization which took over my work and which was directed from then on by individuals inexperienced and incompetent in this type of investigation, has not published a single report on occupational cancers in industry . . . As the result of these delaying and obstructing policies no cancer incidence data of any kind are available on the . . . large worker groups whose members have occupational contact with known or suspected cancer producing chemicals.

During the 1960's, the federal government began to spend huge sums on cancer research; a hurried quest for a cancer cure had begun. Ninety-one million dollars were spent in 1960, $155 million in 1963, and $183 million in 1968. But the carcinogenesis program, focusing on the *causes* of cancer, limped along through this period with a staff of about 100 people and an annual operating budget of less than $2 million. While attention and dollars were being directed to the search for a cancer cure, the carcinogenesis program — the program to identify chemical and physical agents responsible for job-caused cancers — remained the unwanted stepchild of national cancer policy. It remained so because its work — the work of scientists like Hueper — invariably resulted in difficult policy choices. If exposure to uranium ore causes cancer, someone must decide what to do about it. What to do? How to decide? Decisions. Decisions that would frequently impose major costs industrywide and, therefore, directly conflict with the economic interests of many of the nation's most powerful corporations. The easier route was to avoid any controversy by stifling the carcinogenesis program, by shutting off the flow of incriminating evidence.

In 1971, amid great fanfare, President Richard Nixon declared a "war on cancer." In substance, he was proposing more of the same. There would be more research and there would be more money. Much more. The annual budget of the national cancer program, about $200 million in 1971, would swell beyond $500 million within four years, and then to $1 billion before 1980. But the essential direction of the program would remain unchanged. It would continue to follow the path of least resistance — the safest route politically — the search for a cancer cure. No one could properly oppose such a worthy objective. But what of the second dimension to the struggle against cancer? The focus on *causes*? The development of policies to *prevent* exposure to carcinogens, particularly at the workplace? The President did not address these matters.

Discouragingly, current federal policy in the occupational cancer area is only a modest notch or two above the know-nothing/do-nothing policies of the past. In 1970 hopes were temporarily raised among health-conscious reformers when the Congress passed the Occupational Safety and Health Act, an ambitious measure establishing a federal framework for the adoption and enforcement of nationwide occupational health standards. In the laudable words of the Act, its purpose is to assure that "no employee will suffer diminished health, functional capacity, or life expectancy as a result of his work experience." Sponsors of the legislation reasonably believed that the Department of Labor's newly created agency, the Occupational Safety and Health Administration (OSHA), which was to administer the act, would give top priority to setting the toughest possible standards designed to protect workers against job-caused cancer. But throughout 1971, OSHA adopted no new workplace standards. Finally, forced by a legal petition filed by the Industrial Union Department of the AFL-CIO in 1972, OSHA adopted its first cancer-related work standard, a standard for asbestos exposure.

Asbestos. Fifty years ago, who would have believed that this so-called mineral of a thousand uses would one day prove to be a cancer-causing agent with enormous destructive potential? Asbestos is a fibrous silicate mineral that is remarkably effective for insulation and fire-resistance. These qualities have led to its widespread use in shipbuilding, construction work, and in many other industries. Each year, over two billion pounds of asbestos find their way into everyday products. A partial list includes floor tiles, shingles, roofing, wallboard, pipes, potholders, ironing-board covers, electrical insulation tape, filters in gas masks, filters for processing fruit, wine, and pharmaceuticals, plastics, brake linings, clutch facings, carpets, plaster, stucco, cement, and automobile undercoatings. In the words of the writer Paul Brodeur, "There is not an automobile, airplane, train, ship, missile or engine of any sort that does not contain asbestos in some form or another, and it has found its way into literally every building, factory, home, and farm across the land."

Of course, this cornucopia of asbestos products would not be possible without workers. Millions of workers — perhaps as many as five million — are in intimate occupational contact with asbestos. It is not only those who mine, load, truck, and mill the asbestos who breathe and swallow hundreds of millions of microscopic asbestos fibers each workday. Those who work with the milled product are also inhaling and ingesting the fibers — carpenters, insulation workers, heating-equipment workers, rubber workers, asbestos cement makers, putty manufacturers, brake lining producers, roofing and tile manufacturers — the list is almost endless. These are the men and women who, knowingly or unknowingly, risk their lives with their labor because, as it turns out, asbestos is every bit as lethal as it is useful.

British studies dating back to the 1930's established airborne asbestos fibers as a highly dangerous substance. But the studies conducted in the 1960's by Dr. Irving Selikoff of New York's

Mount Sinai Medical Center established, more conclusively, the shocking extent of the danger. Working with New York Local 12 and Newark Local 32 of the International Association of Heat and Frost Insulators and Asbestos Workers, in early 1962 Dr. Selikoff began a major epidemiologic study, one of the great medical detective stories of recent times. Selikoff and his associates pored through the unions' records, obtaining detailed work histories for a sample of 632 men who were on the union rolls as of December 31, 1942. Then they secured the death certificates for those who had died and compared the number of deaths and the causes with those of the general male population of the United States. According to standard mortality tables, 203 deaths could have been expected among the 632 workers. But there were 255, an excess of more than 25 percent. The reason for the excess: cancer. Instead of an expected toll of six or seven deaths from respiratory cancers, there were forty-five. Instead of nine or ten gastrointestinal cancers, there were twenty-nine.

Stated in different terms, Dr. Selikoff found that in the general population, about 18 percent of all Americans die of cancer. Among asbestos insulation workers, the toll approaches 50 percent. Instead of a typical lung cancer rate of 3 or 4 percent, more than 20 percent of all long-term asbestos workers die of respiratory cancer. Instead of an average stomach and colon cancer death rate of 2 or 3 percent, about 6 percent of all long-term asbestos workers succumb to these cancers. Still more die from pleural mesothelioma, an always fatal tumor that attacks the delicate membrane — the pleura — encasing the lungs; or they die from peritoneal mesothelioma, an equally lethal malignancy that attacks the peritoneum — the membrane lining the abdominal cavity. Mesothelioma used to be an exceptionally rare form of cancer. But no longer. About 5 percent of all asbestos workers die from mesothelioma. And case histories indicate that mesothelioma can strike those who had only brief contact with asbestos decades before the cancer actually appeared.

In October of 1972, a forty-seven-year-old financial executive died in a Los Angeles hospital, a victim of pleural mesothelioma. Learning that this malignancy was probably linked to asbestos exposure, the man and his wife used the months before his death to search his background for the origins of the disease. Finally, they hit upon something. In 1944, when he was nineteen years old, the man had worked in a West Coast shipyard for a period of three months. His job was to pack handfuls of asbestos into cloth casings and then pound the casings flat so that they could be wrapped around the miles and miles of steam pipe in warships. Working in a shed, the asbestos dust and fibers filled the air. With each breath he took, millions of tiny, indestructible asbestos fibers lodged in and around his lungs and stomach. Healthy cells, under the stress of this relentless attack, were irreversibly altered and set on a cancerous course. Twenty-seven years after this relatively brief exposure, the mesothelioma appeared in the man's body. Seventeen months later he was dead.

This was no freak incident. It was part of an emerging pattern. Many of those who worked in the shipyards during World War II — young men, housewives, and college coeds who were out of school for the summer — later developed mesotheliomas from asbestos exposures that were of no more than a few weeks' duration. Hearing of these reports, and mindful of the hard data he had himself developed, Dr. Selikoff was so alarmed at the apparent time bomb effect of decades-old asbestos exposures that he estimated that shipyard exposures alone, in the final count, would be seen as the source of many thousands of excess cancer deaths. Asbestos, it appears, is unrivaled as the most pernicious cancer hazard faced by American workers.

Armed with an overwhelming array of evidence, in the spring of 1972, Selikoff and a number of labor union leaders asked the Department of Labor's Occupational Safety and Health Administration to adopt the only prudent policy for dealing with a carcinogen of such demonstrated potency: they urged the adoption of a standard that would progressively cut the permissable levels of airborne asbestos fibers so that, within a few years' time, there would be "no detectable level" of exposure. For their part, industry spokesmen proposed a standard to maintain the status quo.

In the end, on June 6, 1972, OSHA adopted an asbestos

standard that was both peculiar in its construction and disastrous in its impact. The new standard required employers to cut the airborne fiber counts by about one half, thus still allowing workers to inhale many thousands of asbestos fibers with each breath taken. But the reduced exposure level, inadequate as it was, would not take effect for *four* years!

OSHA, an agency originally created to protect the health of workers, had caved in to industry pressure. In effect, the OSHA asbestos standard shunted aside what is perhaps the most fundamental fact of preventive cancer policy: *There is no known "safe level" of exposure to a cancer-causing agent.* A carcinogen is a biologic explosive. It is a bomb with a delayed fuse capable of causing cancer years later among those who were once too near for too long. In 1970, the Ad Hoc Committee on the Evaluation of Environmental Carcinogens, a government-appointed committee whose members were among the nation's most respected cancer researchers, laid this finding before the Congress in the plainest terms. In the committee's words:

> No level of exposure to a chemical carcinogen should be considered toxicologically insignificant for man. For carcinogenic agents a "safe level for man" cannot be established by application of our present knowledge.

The committee called for the progressive elimination of carcinogens from the environment, insisting that the controlling principle must be that human beings have "zero tolerance" to chemical carcinogens.

Quite obviously, OSHA officials were guided by neither scientific nor humanitarian principles. Instead, their compass was political in nature, their goal some kind of a "compromise" on asbestos. But there can be no compromise with carcinogenic exposures. The asbestos standard now in effect is so weak in content that it will have only marginal impact upon the cancer rates among exposed workers. In fact, in a macabre way, it will probably lead to an *increase* in the cancer toll among asbestos workers. For years, asbestos workers have been dying by the thousands from asbestosis — a noncancerous fibrosis or scarring of the lungs. In time, the fibrosis cripples the oxygen-exchange capacity of the lungs, eventually leading to heart failure or death by what amounts to biologic strangulation. To some extent, the reduced exposure levels adopted by OSHA will cut the asbestosis toll. Thirty-year-old asbestos workers, who would have probably died from asbestosis in their fifties, will perhaps escape that disease and live to be sixty or sixty-five, long enough to die instead from asbestos-induced cancer.

Having disposed of the asbestos issue in June 1972, lethargy once again became the top-level policy at OSHA. Months passed without any signs of movement to establish standards for a whole series of known workplace carcinogens. Impatient over the lack of action, in early 1973, the Oil, Chemical, and Atomic Workers Union and Ralph Nader's Washington-based Health Research Group filed a petition with OSHA requesting that exposure levels for ten recognized workplace carcinogens (out of perhaps 100 or more) be set at "zero tolerance"; in other words, there should be no human exposure whatsoever. Even more significantly, the petition included a request that OSHA adopt a precedent-setting permit system that would bar the use of these carcinogens unless a firm first sought and received a government-issued use permit. In this way, a company could not legally use specified cancer-causing substances until OSHA had first surveyed the work environment and certified it to be exposure-free.

A government-issued use permit. A radical concept? Hardly. In principle, a permit system is simply a licensing procedure, the same kind of licensing procedure that has become a fixed feature of American life. Virtually every motor vehicle driver in the United States must secure a license before being allowed to drive an automobile. It is an accepted verity that the government has a legitimate interest in assuring at least a minimum level of competence before allowing an individual to operate an automobile — a potentially lethal instrument. If, in the interest of public safety, nearly 100 million Americans must first secure a driver's license, then surely it is not unreasonable to require the licensing of individual companies in which potent cancer-causing substances are being manufactured or used. That is the essential meaning of a use permit for carcinogens; it provides the leverage of a license to help assure strict adherence to standards designed to prevent job-caused cancer.

In effect, the Oil, Chemical, and Atomic Workers Union and the Health Research Group proposed that their list of ten carcinogens be treated in a way akin to the strict licensing and control provisions placed upon the transportation, manufacture, and use of radioactive materials. And with good reason: the overriding public health hazard is the same — cancer.

One of these ten carcinogens was bis(Chloromethyl)ether, known simply as BCME. BCME is a chemical used in manufacturing resins for water purification and other industrial purposes. Rohm and Haas, a major company, first began using the substance in its Philadelphia plant in the 1940's. In 1962, the company noticed a pattern of lung cancer cases among young men in their thirties, who had worked in one of the buildings. Suspecting that a chemical used only in that building was responsible, by 1967, company-sponsored studies had revealed an increased incidence of lung tumors in both animals and humans breathing BCME; seven workers had already become cancer victims by that time. Despite the installation of better ventilation to reduce exposure to BCME, those workers who had already been exposed to the lethal chemical continued to die, and new workers continued to be exposed. But, throughout this period, the employees were never told that BCME causes cancer. By 1971, the number of lung cancer victims had increased to fourteen. Today, more than a decade after the first signs of an occupational cancer epidemic, Rohm and Haas grudgingly acknowledges more than twenty cancer deaths among exposed workers.

There is more incriminating evidence on BCME from a 1972 field study that the Department of Health, Education and Welfare (HEW) initiated at the Diamond Shamrock Chemical Company in Redwood City, California, just south of San Francisco. Beginning in the mid-1950's, workers in Diamond Shamrock's research and development laboratories were exposed to BCME. No effort was made to contain the BCME exposure until 1966, following the lung cancer deaths of two employees: one, thirty-five years old, the other, forty-eight years old. A year later, a thirty-nine-year-old man, a chemist at the plant, died of lung cancer. In 1971 another worker, thirty-two years old, died from the disease. Then two more workers were struck by lung cancer. All this in a plant that employs about 100 workers. Numbers. Ages. Dates. The human tragedy seems to be lost in the statistical litany. How many more cancer deaths would there be at Diamond Shamrock? How many elsewhere? Recent reports show that BCME — this powerful carcinogen — may be present in a wide range of industrial processes, including the manufacture of permanent press clothing.

Without a permit or licensing system, how can we possibly expect to protect workers from exposure to BCME and other deadly carcinogens? In its strongest form, a permit system would eliminate the expose-now/regrets-later syndrome. Instead, an industry producing or using specified carcinogens would be required to prove that: (1) the substances were essential to its operations; (2) there were no appropriate substitutes of lesser danger; and (3) all necessary steps were being taken to safeguard employees against any exposures whatsoever. The permit system would apply to not only the larger companies like Rohm and Haas and Diamond Shamrock, but also to the smaller outfits like Collins, Caldwell & Dague, where Joe Fitman worked.

On January 29, 1974, OSHA issued its standards for a limited series of carcinogens — the ten listed in the original petition that was filed plus four other carcinogens. There is little comfort in the content of these standards. While OSHA did institute requirements for special handling in the manufacture or use of these fourteen carcinogens, the agency refused to include a requirement insisting that there be "no detectable level" of exposure. In other words, employee exposures to these fourteen cancer-causing substances are still legally permissable. Once again, implicit in OSHA's action was endorsement of the fraudulent notion that there might be a "safe level" of exposure to a carcinogen. In addition to issuing these soft standards, OSHA rejected the all-important permit proposal. The agency made the dubious claim that initiation of such a system was beyond the scope of its statutory authority. But, clearly, what was really involved was a management-oriented aversion to a regulatory framework that would shift the burden of proof to employers and give the benefit of the doubt to workers.

Without a permit system requiring clearance before carcinogens can be produced or used in an individual plant, OSHA will need a veritable army to enforce even the limited standards adopted to date. If, in fact, we are fighting a "war on cancer," then the foremost battlefields must be the workplaces where cancer-causing substances abound. But if this is a war, where are the soldiers? Where are the enforcers of the law, those who safeguard vulnerable employees? Right now, OSHA is little more than a ragtag bureaucracy. It numbers less than 1500 federal occupational health and safety compliance officers. And, of these, fewer than 400 are the more technically qualified industrial hygienists. It's no wonder Joe Fitman couldn't remember ever seeing any health inspectors. With the handful of compliance officers put in the field by OSHA, the odds are good that a small business like Collins, Caldwell & Dague won't be inspected more than once in twenty years.

Who is to blame for the continuing epidemic of job-caused cancer? Industry? In part. Those who recklessly subject employees to carcinogenic exposures cannot escape a major share of the blame. But there should be no illusions about this matter of social and human responsibility. Employers and managers have a mission measured in terms of productivity and profits. There is little room in that equation for considerations of employee health, particularly when the visible damage to health is deferred for many years, as it is with cancer. The assumption, then, must be that employers will do only what they are *required* to do to comply with the law.

But who establishes the requirements of the law? Here is where the larger share of the blame must be placed — on those who make the law and on those who are charged with carrying out its provisions. Those who make the law: the Congress. In 1970, the Congress took an important step forward by enacting the Occupational Safety and Health Act. It is a tough statute that provides ample authority to effectively combat the epidemic of job-caused cancer. But in major matters of regulation the words of a statute alone are not enough; Congress must appropriate the funds necessary to administer the law. This the Congress has failed to do. OSHA's annual budget has hovered around $100 million for several years. One hundred million dollars per year — the amount spent by the Pentagon in just eight hours. OSHA needs at least ten times that much: one billion dollars per year. And it needs the money immediately to hire thousands of inspectors, industrial hygienists, and biostatisticians. The war on cancer must at last be carried into the workplaces across the land. Congress must supply the personnel to inspect the plants and factories and give American workers effective protection against job-caused cancer and other occupational diseases.

Congress can supply the personnel. It can delegate the responsibility. But what about those who are charged with carrying out the law? The Executive Branch. The Nixon and Ford administrations consistently treated the Occupational Safety and Health Act as a nuisance rather than as an opportunity. Their combined record reflects the Executive's systematic unresponsiveness to the problems of job-caused cancer and other job-related health hazards. In fact, these administrations regularly submitted such puny budget projections for OSHA that each year Congress felt obliged to add a few million dollars to the President's embarrassingly inadequate budget requests.

Inadequate budget requests are one way for the Executive to scuttle a program. Another is to appoint officials unworthy of high federal office. From the outset, OSHA's top ranks have been filled by men without distinction, by men who never really believed that the agency had a mission to protect American workers — to save lives. Sometimes their lack of dedication involved more sinister motivations — a kind of malign neglect with predictable consequences. Asbestos was the first round. The standards for fourteen carcinogens was the second round. Standards for dozens of more workplace carcinogens remain to be adopted. But already the pattern has been clearly established: OSHA is both slow and weak, a management-oriented government agency despite its location within the Department of Labor.

Frustrated at the setback on asbestos, and sensing a hidden agenda to sell out American workers, when OSHA finally held public hearings on the question of workplace carcinogens in September 1973, Sheldon Samuels, a spokesman for the AFL-CIO's Industrial Union Department, lashed out at the agency's officials for dragging their feet on the question of cancer-causing substances. Testifying before an OSHA hearing officer he said:

This hearing could have been held more than two years ago . . . The consequence is that, as a result of two years of unjustifiable exposure to carcinogenic agents, regardless of anything done now, hundreds and perhaps thousands of men and women can be expected to experience agonizing death from cancer in the next two decades. Sir, in a truly civilized society we would hold personally responsible those who participated in this crime, both the callous political creatures and the cancer peddlers who bartered moral and statutory obligations. In a just society they would now be undergoing rehabilitation in a penal institution. Instead, they walk freely . . . as if evil is its own reward.

What Samuels suggested was in fact true. There was something far more sinister than ordinary bureaucratic sloth involved here. A year later, in a footnote to the Watergate scandal, it was revealed that OSHA had been thoroughly corrupted during its first fifteen months of operation. In June 1972, instead of being hard at work on standards to protect workers against cancer-causing agents, George C. Guenther, then head of OSHA, was busy drafting a confidential memo to higher-ups in the Department of Labor. In his memo, Guenther assured these administration loyalists that prior to election day "no highly controversial standards will be proposed by OSHA." Eager to use the agency as a prostitute for the Nixon re-election drive, he went on to stress the potential of a management-oriented OSHA as a "sales point for fundraising."

Guenther's betrayal of American workers may not have been the most notorious of the many Watergate crimes, but in time it will certainly prove to be the most deadly.

Part II

Chapter 3.

Pete Gettelfinger

NEW MIDDLETOWN. The name is not fictional. This small town is located in southern Indiana, less than thirty miles from the Kentucky state line. It is a lovely rural setting. Large shade trees and grazing cattle. This is where Raymond "Pete" Gettelfinger, Jr. lived, and where his personal drama was to come to an end. But not before he had a chance to tell the story, in his own words, for all those who cared to listen.

It is November 1974, and Pete Gettelfinger is sitting in the family's seventy-five-year-old, two-story wooden house. He is joined by his wife, Rita. Together, they look like what they are: decent, ordinary, middle-Americans. Rita is seated on a couch with one of their six children. She is a pleasant woman, possessing a buoyant personality. She speaks in a strong voice laced with a distinctive Indiana twang. As for Pete, he's sitting on a wooden rocker. Chemotherapy has caused his hair to fall out, making him look older than his forty-three years. But otherwise, there is nothing in his slim appearance to suggest that he is a dying man. As they sit and speak in the comfort of their home, at times the contradictions seem to border on the bizarre. A fatal disease, yet the appearance of good health. A unique tragedy amid a home environment exuding typicality. By what series of events did a cancer horror story find its way into this household? Pete and Rita Gettelfinger begin to tell the tale.

Rita: For sure this'll be firsthand.

Pete: It will be firsthand. It will be firsthand. I intend to jeopardize no one and to try to get my viewpoint across. We were born and raised, both of us, in Harrison County, Indiana. We were married in New

Middletown up here, half a mile from here. Monday, we will have been married twenty-four years. Yesterday was my forty-third birthday. We have lived on this farm. We have six children. One of 'em works for B. F. Goodrich Company, where I worked for twenty years in the polyvinyl business. He works there now. Well, we've had a real enjoyable life, with the exception of one problem we ran into — angiosarcoma — which has, you might say, changed our life in a tremendous fashion.

Pete Gettelfinger called it "the polyvinyl business." The polyvinyl business. Plastics. It begins with a gas — vinyl chloride. Vinyl chloride was first produced commercially in the United States in 1939. It is an organic chemical, a petroleum-based carbon compound, a gas at room temperature. This colorless gas is fed into large vatlike reactors, eight feet deep and four feet across. The reactors work like industrial pressure cookers. Like magic, they rearrange molecules, converting the vinyl chloride gas into a granular dry resin known as polyvinyl chloride or PVC. It is the PVC resin, sugarlike in appearance, that forms the base for a plethora of solid and flexible plastics: food wrappings, containers, vinyl floor tiles, phonograph records, cups, glasses, dishes, water pipes, toys, car upholstery, tubing and thousands of other commonly used plastic products. A giant American industry has grown up around the discovery of PVC. In the years since commercial production first began, the industry has mushroomed to the point where it now produces more than seven *billion* pounds of polyvinyl chloride a year. Some 300,000 workers are involved in the chain of production: from the synthesis of the gas, to the manufacture of the resin, to the fabrication of the finished plastic products. In 1974, against this backdrop of a spectacular plastics revolution, the industry was compelled to acknowledge that it had what Pete Gettelfinger referred to as "a problem." It had a cancer epidemic in its midst.

The physician at the B. F. Goodrich plant in Louisville is John L. Creech, Jr., a local surgeon. In March 1973, Dr. Creech learned of a case of angiosarcoma of the liver, a malignancy so rare that few doctors see even a single case during a lifetime of practice. But this was the second case he had seen, and both involved polyvinyl chloride workers from B. F. Goodrich. It was a development too ominous to dismiss as mere coincidence. Then, on December 19, 1973, a third patient who had worked at B. F. Goodrich died of angiosarcoma of the liver. Within weeks, the story broke wide open, and the public began to learn of this latest industrial cancer epidemic.

Almost from the beginning, Pete Gettelfinger had been a part of the plastics revolution. He was a participant, a beneficiary, and finally a victim.

I went to work for B. F. Goodrich twenty years ago — in 1954 — because they closed down the power plant where I was working and I needed a job. They put an ad in the paper saying they needed a chemical helper. And I went there and got a job there. I was a chemical helper there. That involved primarily cleaning up the polymerizers. In different places you've seen them written down as reactors or pots. They're polymerizers is what they are. They're high-pressured tanks which will control reactions taking place in them.

In regard to the cleaning of the reactors, which has been an issue throughout the vinyl chloride problem . . . you have a residue build-up on the wall of your reactor and in some cases you have a water residue in the bottom. And that, when I went to work there, that was the job of the helper — to get in and take the residue off the inside wall of the reactor, which we done with scrapers. And if there was any build-up that was left on the bottom, we'd pick it up and bring it out. Now, we had to pull out the excess vinyl chloride vapor in order for us to survive in there. When I began we wore nothing for protection. All we done was took an exhaust hose and stuck it in there and sucked the vinyl chloride gas out and we got in. We didn't wear anything except the clothes we wore.

Vinyl chloride is a heavy gas — much heavier than air — and it will settle close to the bottom. Now, vinyl chloride has a characteristic that if there should be a mixture near the bottom of the vessel or reactor you were in, your feet would start feelin' cold if there was much in there. Then you would know it was time to get out of there and see what is wrong. That, in the early years when I worked there, that was your first warning sign — your feet. Vinyl chloride will tell you on your feet.

Now, the residue on the wall after your reaction — you'd chip it off the walls and it'd fall to the bottom. And you'd pick it out with your hands in a five-gallon bucket or a three-gallon bucket. Bare hands or leather gloves, primarily leather gloves. And your hands were wet. Your hands were wet. In some of them reactors the temperature gets hot. In the summertime I've seen it when I know it was 120 degrees. It was hot. Real hot. We were expected to clean five reactors in an eight-hour shift. We'd run anywhere from forty-five minutes to an hour and fifteen minutes depending on how they come down, whether they come down real clean or bad — it depends on the reaction. We would have one man looking in the reactor and one man inside. Definitely the harder work would be inside. Actually, the work was so hard while we were in there that we wouldn't put in as many hours as we would in our normal day. When we were in there, we were doing as hard labor as a man has had to do — as hard as I've done. And I've done plenty of hard labor working on a farm.

In the early years, we didn't know we were dealing with a dangerous substance. Our two main things were explosion and fire. That's what we worry about. You can ask my wife or any other man's wife. They never — nobody ever thought about anything but if there'd be an explosion there or a fire. That was what we worried about, 'cause one spark could do as much damage as if you'd brought a blow torch in there. That was our primary concern up until this business that's been gettin' to us. Something serious. Something that is costing — has cost — some of our lives.

"Something serious. Something that is costing — has cost — some of our lives." Liver cancer. Situated under the right rib cage, the liver is a large organ, weighing three to four pounds in an adult. So vital is the organ to the maintenance of life — storing carbohydrate, manufacturing plasma protein, and removing drugs and poisons from the blood — that nearly all of the 10,000 Americans each year who are diagnosed for liver cancer are dead within twelve months. Cancers that begin in the liver — primary liver cancers — have become more common in recent years, accounting for about 1 in 40 of all malignancies. But the particular liver tumor that Pete Gettelfinger and other vinyl chloride workers had was anything but common. Called angiosarcoma, this tumor attacks the blood vessels deep within the liver, disabling the organ, ultimately strangling it. Historically, angiosarcoma of the liver has been so rare that there have been fewer than thirty cases per year reported throughout the entire United States.

On the afternoon of March 1, 1974 — after a surgical biopsy — Pete Gettelfinger knew for sure that he had angiosarcoma of the liver. The news was depressing but not surprising. In the months preceding surgery, there had been multiple tests, and the results were pointing to the worst possibilities. In addition, there was the logic of the unfolding tragedy: Pete's work history spanned two decades of involvement with virtually every phase of the PVC production process. He was regularly breathing heavy concentrations of vinyl chloride gas — 200 parts per million (ppm), 500 ppm, 1000 ppm, and even 5000 ppm. Then, too, there were those worrisome recollections — flashbacks to the mid-1960's when the workers began to express an uneasiness about the early deaths among their colleagues.

I feel that the men were aware that something was wrong. We just got to noticin' that there was just a few too many of us young men — see, the men working in the company, we were young men. They were losin' too many guys. As we sat and ate and had our breaks, we just got to thinkin' that maybe there might be a little too much — too many of us guys just gettin' out of this world too young.

We just talked about it, I'd say, in general conversation. General conversation. Very little was done. There were people who would say something's wrong. Perhaps at one time or another I said it — I can't recall specifically if I said it. But there was something wrong — just too many of us gettin' in trouble. It seemed like there was too many of the young guys dyin' compared to what we would see in other areas.

Rita: Well, it was in November of 1973 that they — well maybe the later part of October — that they had done his first test. But it was in November when he came home and told me that one of his first tests had come back with something on it. And it was a hard word to say. And you thought — well, I think my thoughts were — I kept thinkin' that well, well it can't be. And we didn't mention it. We didn't say anything to the kids about it. And then it was probably the first part of January or so that WHAS had an item on their newscast about it. They had — you know —

they were discussin' this possibility that there could be an outbreak of liver cancer at Goodrich. And they thought they had found some. So we were sittin' here watchin' the news and one of the children turned around to their daddy and says: "Are you one of 'em?"

Pete: Well, I didn't feel bad. At that time, I didn't feel bad. Two of my liver function tests did not look good, so they decided to get me out of the vinyl chloride building. And Dr. Creech said, "Ray," he said, "I'm going to put you in the hospital." The last day I worked was the 22nd of February, and they put me in the hospital on the 23rd.

Rita: He went to work then on a Monday, and he came into the office where I work about ten o'clock and told me they were going to have to take a look at his liver. And I think it's one of these things — no matter how well you think you're prepared . . .

Pete: On March 1 they operated on me. An exploratory operation. And after the operation the first thing that I knew was when Dr. Creech came down to me in the recovery room and he said, "Well, I'm sorry to tell you that you have angiosarcoma."

I made up my mind, before they took me to the operating room, whatever will be will be and I will accept it. I will accept whatever they might discover. I prepared myself for it bein' real good and I prepared myself for it bein' real bad. It turned out, in the eyes of most, to be real bad. No, I wouldn't say that. I'd say it turned out, in the eyes of most, to be impossible. In my opinion it was real bad. But I still think I've got a chance.

Rita: I kept tellin' myself the day that we were sittin' there — they took him to surgery about eleven o'clock and it was about three-thirty before Dr. Creech came back. And I mean no matter how you tell yourself that I'm ready for this — I sort of thought, you know, well, I'm going to be like the Rock of Gibraltar no matter what comes. Well, the Rock of Gibraltar sort of crumbled. But to be able to say how I felt — when Dr. Creech finished talking with us I had the very definite feeling that my whole world had absolutely collapsed around me. But, yet, being the mother of six children you turn around and look and you think: maybe that world hasn't collapsed around me. One portion of my world has collapsed around me. But should something happen to him, I have got a much bigger job on my hands than I have right now.

After the exploratory surgery and confirmation of angiosarcoma, Pete Gettelfinger became the center of a medical saga. Because of what his case represented — a prototype of perhaps many hundreds of vinyl chloride–induced cancers yet to appear — it was decided to begin a program of treatment and observation at the National Institutes of Health Hospital in Bethesda, Maryland. Every week or two Pete boarded the 8:00 A.M. Eastern Airlines jet from Louisville to Washington, D.C. and then took a twenty-minute taxi ride to Bethesda, Maryland. Once in Bethesda, he underwent scores of tests and examinations. And then chemotherapy — the administration of powerful anticancer drugs to slow or perhaps temporarily halt the liver cancer's spread.

The air shuttle to Bethesda and back took on the character of a prayerful pilgrimage. Medical science became the newly adopted faith; the NIH Hospital became the house of worship. At the NIH Hospital, Pete was the object of intense study by a host of national and international cancer specialists. Implicit in their heroics was a desperate search for hope. Not just for Pete Gettelfinger and his family, but for the others — their names still unknown — who, as a result of exposure to vinyl chloride, had suffered irreversible cell damage and were destined to develop malignancies.

For the Gettelfinger family, the task was adjustment — adjusting to the ups and downs, the momentary glimmers of hope.

Pete: My tumor is in my liver about right here [pointing to the right rib cage]. *And, its size is just about the size of these two grapes here, shaped about like a bean. It's got a curve in the middle. Now, one of their major considerations is whether to operate. My situation has not changed noticeably in the last few months. That is one route — to operate and try to take the tumor out. Or, chemotherapy, to just see if we can deal with it. I know that they're doin' their best. And I know that there's many of 'em workin' on it. The more of 'em that there are workin' on it, the better the chance of a successful solution. I'd go back there to Bethesda on Eastern Airlines tonight if I knew for sure that they'd have some definite thing in the morning, because suspense is actually now beginning to get to us. The suspense is beginning to get to all of us now. It's been getting too high. But I still maintain my confidence. I've got the best doin' their best. What else could they do?*

Rita: When we were in Bethesda, the chaplain — he'd come and talk to him a lot and he would come talk to me and so on — and he was talkin' about all the faith and hope and the confidence that Pete had, you know. And I just laughed and said, "Well, why do you think you see me in mass every morning? Because," I says, "I don't have all that faith and hope or confidence." And he said, "Well, don't feel bad about it." And I said, "Well, I feel like I've got to go and be revitalized every day!"

Pete: It gets to you once in a while.

From the beginning, Pete's ordeal was a shared experience, shared by family and the general community, but shared in a special way by those who worked with him. His coworkers were compelled to live in the shadow of this cancer epidemic. And so an intimate comaraderie took hold. Angiosarcoma, they were told, is a fatal liver cancer. There are no survivors. But maybe Pete would change that. Maybe the pilgrimage to Bethesda would produce a cancer cure or, at least, an effective treatment. Something. Some kind of hedge against the cancer pox.

Pete: I took pride in the kind of work I was doing. Definitely. Definitely. Definitely. 'Cause I can say this myself: from the raw material on the loading stations, all the way to sending the finished product out, I have done all those things. I've seen it done good and I've seen it done bad . . .

You know, every one of the men who's died so far, I knew. All of those who died were friends. Every one of those men I knew well. Every one of those men I knew well. Two of 'em I worked with from the first day I went to work there. They had angiosarcoma. I worked with them half my life.

Rita: It sort of sends a chill up and down your back. I mean, every one of them he had either been to their funeral or to the funeral home to see them.

Pete: Before I knew I had it. Before I knew I had it. That's right. They were friends of mine I'd worked with a long time. And your friendship is a little closer there.

Rita: I think that was proven by the number of men that he worked with that came to Saint Anthony's Hospital to see him when he had his biopsy.

Pete: You know they waited in line.

Rita: I mean there was, you know, every day there was quite a number of them.

Pete: Over the period of eight months, most of 'em have made a point to contact me in one way or another. And not to be nosy, either.

Waiting it out. Having to stare at the reality of an untimely death under unlikely circumstances. When forced to confront the prospect of their own premature demise, people tend to turn to larger themes, trying to establish some kind of understanding about their fate. In Pete's case the thoughts were of Hope and Purpose and Moral Responsibility.

Hope:

My weight's held good, and I think I've got the finest crew of doctors in the world workin' on it. And I've had certain groups of chemotherapy which is why I'm losin' my hair. Incidentally, I've got back some of it and started growin' a mustache two or three days ago just to show I mean business! I still have confidence in my doctors. I get a complete physical exam every time out there — perhaps more than most people do. The burden is not as hard on me as it is on those around me. I know that.

I will say that they — my family — have been tough. But how tough you have to be under the circumstances is awful tough. It's hurt 'em. It's hurt 'em. They have backed me up beautifully, but it's hurt 'em. They've had to be tougher than I have — much — because I know what my situation is. And I would almost say that almost any of 'em would be willing to take my place . . . Everyone else — most guys didn't have a chance. They didn't have a chance. I know the odds are bad but not as bad as they were before, because I've already done better than the other fellas. We've done better than those preceding us, because they didn't have any chance at all. And right now I think we've got a heck of a good chance. I think we have awakened the medical and petrochemical industry to the extent that they will provide the very best they can. And perhaps we might — through me or someone else — we might find something that will cure some cancers for many fellas. There's been lots of money spent on me to try to cure me. I know that.

Right now I'm expectin' to go back to Maryland in a week or two. Right now I'm taking no medicine at all. No chemotherapy. Right now the doctors are deciding what to do next. I leave it up to the judgment of the good doctors, and I'm hopin' that one of 'em or all of 'em know what they're doing. Oh, I've got confidence in 'em. If I didn't have any confidence in 'em, I wouldn't have lasted this long. I don't see how anyone could.

Rita: A lot of people will say, "I don't see how you do it." And, I mean, my thought immediately is: Well, what are our choices? Please pitch me out some choices. We might want to grab one of those! But, I mean, I think that when we all get together, I guess maybe there's a safety in numbers. We feel like we can, you know, sort of whip the world when we're all together.

I really think one of the hardest things for me — and it sounds awful, and I mean I really appreciate people's concern — but it's the fact that people keep askin' you over and over again — every day. And, I mean, you just wish — you appreciate it but yet you just wish that they would let you forget it for just . . . But I think that my supervisor — with the highway department — he pretty well summed it up. He said, "Look," he says, "I don't come in every day and ask you about it." He says, "That doesn't mean that I'm not thinkin' about it. But," he says, "when I come into the office and I see you sittin' there workin', I think maybe just for an instant she has put it in the back of her mind." He said, "There is no point in me stoppin' and bringing it up."

Pete: We've had many people come by. And I'll tell you something. There are so many people been so dern good to us that . . .

Rita: And the number of people you will meet that will say, "We're prayin' for you." And, if nothing else, it really reinstates your faith in humanity. And, I mean, these are people that — you can tell — they really mean it. I mean it's not just a bunch of loose words. They really mean it.

Purpose:

Pete: I think about this a lot — it's helped me a whole lot — the fact that we got 6500 guys in the United States makin' a livin' workin' with

*polyvinyl chloride in the form I was usin' it in. And I'll bet you we've got
a million that are makin' a livin' in plastics. And I feel that our industry
must survive. I think our industry must survive. And, I'll cite to you an
example. The whole petrochemical industry is now maybe fifty years old,
just since they made their first little thing. And the plastics industry, you
might say is thirty or thirty-five years old. And it has economically given
millions of people things that they couldn't have. If it wasn't for plastics,
now, the price of wood would be so expensive that the average man
couldn't afford to have a rockin' chair like this one on where I'm settin'.
And, yet, that's killin' people. It may kill me. Look how much safer it's
made an automobile or the wiring in your home. Look at the safety features that's put in the home. So far now they only got twenty-eight dead
[worldwide]. And they got two or three they don't know what's goin' to
happen to them. But the industry is tremendously important. That's why
it's so important for the industry to survive — for the employees that work
with it. You've got to look at everyone's viewpoint. I can't say that I'm one
of the lucky guys, but I must say that as long as we have put products on
the market that has helped the average person economically — that must
be weighed against all that's bad too.*

Moral Responsibility:

*I have no bitterness toward any individual. But I don't think that the
petrochemical industry, from the beginning, did the best they could. I
don't think they did the best they could. But to pinpoint an individual —
like the plant manager or three or four of them — no. But I think that
nationally and internationally — I don't think they did the best they
could. Now, there's some reasons there. You see they began — you might
say it was during World War II — these companies were filling these war
orders and they got to the point where some of the basic things were just let
go, 'cause we had to have a product and we had to have it now. I think
that was one of the basic reasons that maybe they didn't do as much as they
could have otherwise. And how long anybody knew that there was a
cancer danger before I was told I had it? I don't know. But I suspect that
someone knew up there for a while, somewhere in the industry, 'cause they
had a product and they were sellin' it. You think about it. A year ago,
angiosarcoma — the average man never heard of it. Too much has
turned up too quick. But so far as any personal animosity toward any
man or any part of management — I have none that I can locate, and I*

prefer never to locate it. Because it's comforting to not have any bitterness. But I'm afraid maybe somebody might have knew something before they . . .

Rita: But if they did, you have to go back to the old theory that every man has been appointed one day to answer. And if he knew and didn't do anything about it, he's going to have to answer.

Pete: But we don't bear any grudges. Anyhow, I have waited eight months and I know no more now than I did when Dr. Creech told me I had angiosarcoma. Except, I know that it hasn't gotten any worse. And, on the bills, the company and I have got along fine so far. They have a problem and I have one.

Rita: I'm a little biased, but I think our problem's a little bigger than theirs!

Pete: Yeah, but suppose you were the biggest stockholder in the company though?

Rita: But I think that — I mean — you don't want to give up hope. But yet on the other hand I have tried to look at it from the aspect of now, you know, suppose we aren't successful. And, I mean, I don't mean to be despairing but, yet, we have six children, one youngster that's only eleven and one that's fourteen. And, I mean, there's a lot of things to consider. It gets a little hard to take — to sit and watch the newscast, and they talk about fatal liver disease. But I think this has been true of all of us. We have — sort of like a yo-yo — we go up and down. We have our good times and we have our bad times. We have all been down the road step by step.

By the time Pete Gettelfinger died, he had become something of a local and a national celebrity in his grim struggle against cancer. On March 19, 1975, *The Corydon Democrat,* a newspaper serving southern Indiana, reported his funeral with a front page headline:

"PETE" GETTELFINGER BURIED SATURDAY IN NEW MIDDLETOWN

It was a cool, bright, almost spring-like day Saturday when Raymond P. (Pete) Gettelfinger Jr., perhaps a victim of the Industrial Age, was laid to rest in a little cemetery in New Middletown.

Gettelfinger, 43, died Tuesday evening, March 11, at St. Anthony's Hospital in Louisville . . .

Gettelfinger is the sixth worker at the B. F. Goodrich Co. plant on Bells Lane in Louisville to die of angiosarcoma . . .

A year ago in February, doctors told Gettelfinger that he had the disease. He was placed on retirement disability, and he began getting chemotherapy treatments at the National Institutes of Health in Bethesda, Md. . . .

Despite his optimism and faith, Gettelfinger's condition gradually worsened and he entered St. Anthony's on January 26. He was placed in isolation for protection because his weakened body had lost its ability to resist germs. He died at 9:55 P.M. on March 11. He had been in a coma for about a week.

Prayers were said at a wake service Friday night at the Gehlbach-Royse Funeral Home in Corydon. After Gettelfinger died, nearly 1000 people visited the funeral home to pay their respects.

Chapter 4.

Human Test Animals

AT THE OFFICE OF OCCUPATIONAL HEALTH SURVEILLANCE AND BIOMETRICS in Rockville, Maryland, government officials have established a running account of reported cases of liver angiosarcoma among workers exposed to vinyl chloride or polyvinyl chloride. The cases are summarized on a statistical table where they are neatly numbered. Pete Gettlefinger is no. 09. His birthdate is recorded: 11-08-31. His date of first exposure to vinyl chloride: 09-09-54. The date of diagnosis for angiosarcoma: 03-01-74. Throughout 1975, under the category "date of death," the word "ALIVE" appeared. In the spring of 1975, the data on case no. 09 were revised. The word "ALIVE" was removed and the date of death was dutifully recorded: 03-11-75.

When Pete Gettelfinger died, there were fifteen reported cases of vinyl chloride-induced liver cancer in the United States. Early in 1976, the number had grown to nineteen. The count goes on. And on. And on. Since the latent period from first exposure to the date of a cancer diagnosis has ranged from eleven to thirty years, the final death toll from pre-1975 exposures to vinyl chloride won't be known until after the year 2000. But this much seems certain: the deaths will reach up into the hundreds by then, perhaps even into the thousands. In all likelihood, in the decades ahead, the federal government's Office of Occupational Health Surveillance and Biometrics will continue to maintain the lengthening record of vinyl chloride deaths. No doubt this record will be of some value to cancer statisticians. But, placed in the larger context of the cancer pox, the government's effort is really a pitiful throwback to the same kinds of primitive body counts that have always characterized occupational cancer epidemics. Two centuries ago, Dr. Percival Pott counted the chimney sweeps dead from scrotal cancer. In the late 1800's, Dr. Ludwig Rehn counted German dyestuff workers dying from bladder cancer. And in this century, among chromate workers and uranium miners, Dr. Hueper counted the dead bodies consumed by lung cancer. Must occupational cancer policy begin and end with after-the-fact, body-count bookkeeping? Absolutely not. There *is* a better way, a proven technique of cancer prevention utilizing what are known as bioassays.

Bioassays. Bioassays for carcinogenic activity. Simply stated, bioassays to determine carcinogenic activity involve the use of animals — usually small rodents such as rats, mice, or hamsters — to test the cancer-causing properties of chemical compounds. Vinyl chloride offers an excellent example of how valuable bioassays can be. In 1970, in Bologna, Italy, Dr. Cesare Maltoni began a series of experiments administering vinyl chloride gas to hundreds of laboratory rats. His work proceeded in utmost secrecy, without the knowledge of any government, and known only to a handful of corporate officials who had commissioned the work on behalf of a consortium of major chemical companies. To carry out his experiments, Maltoni carefully divided the rats into groups. For example, in one experiment he divided nearly 500 rats into half a dozen groups. In enclosed chambers, he administered doses of vinyl chloride so that for four hours a day, five days a week, some of the rats were inhaling 10,000 ppm of the chemical; others 6000 ppm, 2500 ppm, 500 ppm, and 250 ppm. One control group received no vinyl chloride exposure at all. After 127 weeks in the exposure chambers, Maltoni removed the rats and let them live out the remaining months of their lives. When they died, an autopsy was performed on each, with a careful examination of tissue samples from the lungs, kidneys, spleen, liver, brain, and other vital organs.

The results were horrifying. Of the sixty-nine animals exposed to 10,000 ppm of vinyl chloride, six developed liver angiosarcomas. Of the seventy-two animals exposed to 6000 ppm, eleven developed the disease. At 2500 ppm, nine of seventy-four rats succumbed to liver angiosarcoma. At 500 ppm, seven of sixty-seven developed the fatal malignancy. And at 250 ppm, two of sixty-seven died from the disease. At the same time, Maltoni's control group of animals — rats that were kept in chambers without any exposure to vinyl chloride gas — did not develop any cases of liver angiosarcoma. The results underscored two key points: first, vinyl chloride is a potent carcinogen, even when administered in relatively low doses; and, second, vinyl chloride exhibits the same kind of general dose-response relationship common to cancer-causing substances. In other words, the higher the dose, the higher the incidence of malignant tumors. Conversely, the lower the dose, the lower the incidence of malignant tumors.

By the fall of 1972, Maltoni had seen enough to be absolutely convinced. In reporting preliminary results to his sponsors, he said the bioassays really constituted a prediction. A prediction of a likely cancer epidemic among vinyl chloride workers. As it turned out, scarcely months later, Maltoni's prediction began to emerge as reality: like Maltoni's rats, vinyl chloride workers who had incurred long-term exposures to the gas were succumbing to liver cancer at a rate more than sixteen times normal; and, like the dose-response relationship exhibited among Maltoni's rats, those workers exposed to the substance in the greatest quantities — regularly inhaling vinyl chloride concentrations ranging up into the hundreds of parts per millions — were at greatest risk.

In one sense, the vinyl chloride tragedy teaches an old lesson of the biologic link between test animals and humans. But the tragedy teaches more than this. It teaches a lesson about deadly negligence, governmental and corporate negligence, in failing to apply available scientific methods to test carcinogens in the industrial environment. Consider again Maltoni's work. It involved approximately 500 rodents in a controlled study administered by an able scientist. The total time: approximately three years. The total cost: roughly $100,000. Measured against the multibillion-dollar resources of the plastics industry, the outlay for the carcinogenesis bioassay on vinyl chloride amounts to little more than petty cash. Yet, the animal testing on vinyl chloride was not begun until 1970, even though the techniques to determine a substance's cancer-causing potential were available long before Maltoni commenced his work. In fact, carcinogenesis bioassays date back to the early part of this century. In 1908, a Frenchman named Clunet induced cancer among rats by deliberately exposing them to x-rays. In 1915, two Japanese investigators, Yamagiwa and Ichikawa, produced skin cancer in rabbits by applying coal tar to their ears every two or three days. And here, in the United States, Hueper induced bladder cancer in dogs by administering beta-Naphthylamine, since recognized as a chief agent in causing bladder cancer among dye workers. Why, then, when the mass production of polyvinyl chloride began in 1939 had there been no pretesting of vinyl chloride gas to determine its cancer-causing effects on animals and, therefore, its potential threat to workers? The answer seems to be that pretesting for carcinogenesis wasn't done simply because it wasn't required by the federal government. It wasn't required in 1939. Nor was it required in 1949. Or 1959. Or 1969. Or 1975.

Beginning in 1971, the Congress had before it a proposed Toxic Substances Control Act, legislation that would establish regulatory machinery to require animal testing of thousands of chemical compounds already widely used and also pretesting of chemical compounds not yet in commercial use. These bioassays would be designed to determine not only a substance's cancer-causing properties but also its capacity to cause birth defects, mutations, and poisoning. Despite the vinyl chloride horror story, the Toxic Substances Control Act languished in Congress amid relentless industrial pressure, particularly from chemical companies determined to kill the bill outright or to hopelessly dilute its key provisions.

The reasoned statements of eminent cancer researchers seemed to have little impact upon Congress. Dr. Umberto Saffiotti, until recently the National Cancer Institute's Associate Director for Carcinogenesis, presented the essentials of the case in 1972:

> [A number of] chemical substances have been shown to be carcinogenic by tests in animals . . . Several individual chemicals or mixtures of chemicals have also been shown conclusively to be carcinogenic

by direct observation in man . . . With the exception of arsenic, still under experimental study, all the main products that were found to be carcinogenic by direct evidence in man have also been proven carcinogenic in animals. On the other hand, proof that a substance, which had been recognized as carcinogenic in animals, actually causes cancer in man would require, in most cases extremely complex and lengthy epidemiologic studies . . . Therefore, the only prudent course of action at the present state of our knowledge is to assume that chemicals which are carcinogenic in animals could also be so in man, although the direct demonstration in man is lacking.

There is more to the argument for pretesting. Consider the time bomb effect of the long latent period associated with carcinogens. As Dr. Saffiotti explained:

The fact that it may take twenty years to detect in man the cancers due to the exposure to a new chemical carcinogen means that the chemical can be given to people for 20 years under the false appearance of harmlessness. If the effect is then detected and properly attributed to the specific chemical, and this is then removed from the environment, the cancers it induced will continue to appear for the next 20 to 30 years.

Saffiotti used the lesson of thalidomide to emphasize the point:

Now let us assume that thalidomide, instead of producing deformities which are readily detected in a matter of months when the babies are born, produced a form of cancer, which would only become manifest when babies grow into adults. The lethal effects of the drug would probably still be undetected . . . Women would possibly still be taking it during pregnancy, and a large number of people would have been born with a built-in sentence to early death by cancer.

But what of the argument that a rodent is not a man and, therefore, that a substance that induces cancer in animals will not necessarily do so in humans? It is, of course, possible that a substance causing cancer in a rodent will not do so in humans. It is possible, yes. But the overwhelming body of evidence points to a strong correlation between a carcinogen's impact on test animals and its impact on humans. Vinyl chloride is only the latest example.

But what of those instances where a substance appears to be

only mildly carcinogenic in animals? Perhaps it causes only a few tumors among several hundred test animals and, even then, only when high doses of the carcinogen are administered. Is this real cause for concern? It should be. Since carcinogenesis bioassays can merely serve as a rough approximation of what the human experience may be, it is important to remember that the human experience may prove far *worse* than the animal experience. In other words, a chemical agent may be only mildly carcinogenic in a population of test animals but highly carcinogenic in the exposed human population. For example, it was with considerable difficulty that researchers finally demonstrated the cancer-causing effects of certain aniline dyes in test animals. But dye workers with long-term exposures were succumbing to bladder cancer at rates that, in some instances, approached 100 percent. Obviously, aniline dyes were far more carcinogenically reactive in human tissue than in the tissue of certain animal species.

The comparative complexity of the human body and its exposure to a myriad of environmental agents that may actually enhance a carcinogen's impact suggest that there may be many instances where a carcinogen portends far greater consequences in the human population than might be indicated by a mildly positive impact upon animals. Despite this biologic fact of life, there will always be those who confidently predict that a substance won't cause cancer in humans though it does in animals. Given our state of knowledge at this point, no one is wise enough to be able to make such a prediction. And those who pretend to be are either engaging in a wildly dangerous fantasy or they are simply doing the bidding of corporate interests with a stake in selling the public on the "safety" of a cancer-causing substance. Dr. Saffiotti's words bear repeating, for they are the basis upon which future cancer policy must be built.

. . . The only prudent course of action at the present state of our knowledge is to assume that chemicals which are carcinogenic in animals would also be so in man, although the direct demonstration in man is lacking.

If the usefulness of carcinogenesis bioassays was not obvious thirty-five years ago, there is no escaping their necessity now. It comes down to a matter of self-preservation in a chemicalized society. The petrochemical revolution, which spawned vinyl chloride in 1939, has since accelerated to the point where each year literally thousands of new chemical compounds are developed. And, of these, several hundred are destined to enter industrial and commercial channels, most of them untested for their cancer-causing properties. At this moment the backlog of chemicals that should be bioassayed for their carcinogenicity runs into the tens of thousands. Yet, only about 1000 have been properly tested for their cancer-causing potential. The magnitude of a first carcinogenesis screening of the environment — involving perhaps 20,000 or more chemicals — is staggering. But it is staggering only because the neglect has itself been of a staggering magnitude.

It is important to stress that the problem, huge as it is, is not hopeless. A law to prevent the marketing of any *new* chemicals that have not been pretested for carcinogenesis is a long overdue first step, effectively placing a moratorium on the mindless proliferation of new chemicals that are untested for their cancer-causing properties. The second step, perhaps taken in the context of a ten-year plan, should be the legally required carcinogenesis testing of chemical compounds *already* in use. Those most widely used or those suspect for their cancer-causing potential should be screened first. The cost of this undertaking might run as high as $2 billion, spread over a decade. Two billion dollars in ten years. Two hundred million dollars per year. The cost is both reasonable and manageable. Measured against chemical industry sales that exceeded $72 *billion* in 1975, or against after-tax profits that exceeded $5.5 *billion,* $200 million a year in testing costs is not nearly as large a sum as it first appears. Moreover, since the costs, by law, are to be borne by the firms seeking to market and profit from the chemical substance, the expenses involved in carcinogenesis testing would simply become an added cost of doing business. In the parlance of the Internal Revenue Code, an "ordinary and necessary business expense"; a deductible item that, in the end, may, or may not, be reflected in a fractional increase in the retail cost of the product.

So much for costs. What about benefits? Mandatory carcinogenesis testing buys the kind of baseline data — a carcinogenesis inventory — essential to a rational and effective policy of cancer prevention. In cancer prevention, the earlier the intervention the greater the payoff. History has offered examples to underscore this point. In 1940, promoters of a new pesticide, N-2-fluorenylacetamide or 2-FAA for short, sought to market the compound throughout the United States. Researchers, who were conducting routine toxicity tests simply to determine the poisoning capacity of the substance, discovered that 2-FAA is a powerful carcinogen, causing a wide spectrum of malignancies in test animals. Tumors. Tumors everywhere. Tumors of the liver. Tumors of the breast. Tumors of the bladder and kidney. Tumors of the lung. As a result of this accidental discovery, 2-FAA was never marketed, and the American people were spared what may have become a cancer epidemic. Ironically, 2-FAA is utilized today on a limited basis by cancer researchers. They find the substance helpful to their study of cancer precisely because of its sure-fire capacity to produce malignant tumors at multiple sites in test animals.

Another example of the value of carcinogenesis bioassays emerged in 1969. Under a contract with the National Cancer Institute, a firm called Bionetics Research Laboratories completed carcinogenesis bioassays on 120 separate industrial compounds and pesticides. Eleven produced tumors in test animals; 109 did not. These results were important in two respects: first, in identifying eleven substances known to cause cancer in animals — the most notable being DDT — it became impossible for government policymakers to ignore the cancer hazards that these specific carcinogens posed to humans; and, second, these bioassays identified a number of chemical substances that appeared to be free of cancer-causing properties. One hundred nine of 120 substances tested proved to be apparently "clean." This was not unusual. Contrary to the false and fatalistic notion that "everything causes cancer," the fact is that the vast majority of industrial and commercial substances are *not* carcinogenic. Out of 20,000 or more environmentally significant substances, those that produce cancer probably number no more than several hundred. The real challenge, then, is the same as it has been for decades: to identify the agents that are carcinogenic in animals and then to adopt and enforce the strictest preventive measures to eliminate or, at least minimize, human exposure to these substances.*

Prevention must become the guidepost of national cancer policy. The logic of prevention is irrefutable. The cancerization process almost always follows the same chain of events. The first link: a carcinogen is introduced into the occupational or general environment. The second link: the carcinogen enters the human body. The third link: it penetrates into target cells. The fourth link: the target cells are transformed into malignant cells. The fifth link: the malignant cells multiply and grow into a tumor. Interruption of this chain of events at any point may lead to the successful control of a cancer. But the most promising method of control — the surest and the most humane — is to use carcinogenesis bioassays to break the chain of cancerization at the very first link, at the point where the carcinogen is about to be introduced into the occupational or general environment. That is the essence of toxic substances control legislation.

Finally, after years of tragic delay, on September 28, 1976, Congress adopted the Toxic Substances Control Act. On October 12, the President signed the measure into law. But, as with the Occupational Safety and Health Act, statutory language alone is not enough. Its implementation cannot be left to reluctant administrators. The President must see to it that the men

---

*A recent breakthrough may make it possible to be much more efficient in screening chemical agents than has historically been the case. The Ames test, named after its developer, Professor Bruce Ames of the University of California at Berkeley, provides a cheap and quick indication of a chemical's cancer-causing potential by its observed effect on bacteria. Requiring only a few days to perform, the Ames test is based on the fact that nearly all chemicals that cause cancer in animals and man also produce mutations in bacterial cultures. Therefore, agents found to be mutagenic in bacteria must be regarded as suspect carcinogens. Important as it is, the Ames test is not a substitute for animal testing, but rather offers a valuable means of selecting those agents for which long-term carcinogenesis testing — in live animals — must begin immediately.

and women recruited to the Environmental Protection Agency — the agency charged with principal responsibility for implementing the Toxic Substances Control Act — are unswervingly committed to fulfilling its protective intent. Moreover, the President must assure the personal political support necessary to secure adequate congressional funding of all phases of the act. To do anything less would be a fraud upon the American people.

Beyond the imperative of carcinogenesis bioassays, there are other lessons to be learned from the vinyl chloride calamity. On August 21, 1974, seven months after the vinyl chloride cancer link was first disclosed to the public, the Congress heard a report on the government's action as of that date. Dr. Joseph Wagoner, then Director of Field Studies and Clinical Investigations of the National Institute for Occupational Safety and Health (NIOSH), testified that his agency had organized a field study to determine the nature and extent of the cancer epidemic at the B. F. Goodrich plant in Louisville. The results were shocking. Even at that early date, before additional cases had been diagnosed, NIOSH reported that the men in the Goodrich plant were dying from liver cancer at eleven times the expected rate. But there was more. They were dying at extraordinary rates from other less exotic kinds of cancers, too. They were dying from brain cancer at five and one-half times the normal rate; dying from lymphoma and leukemia at nearly two times the expected rate; and dying from cancer of the lung and respiratory system at one and one-half times the expected rate. What NIOSH confirmed, then, was that B. F. Goodrich's Louisville operation was the focus of a full-blown, in-plant cancer epidemic. The confirmation came in August 1974. But the same kind of systematic survey, had it been conducted years earlier — perhaps as early as the mid-1960's — could have documented the epidemic in its incipient stages. As Pete Gettelfinger recalled:

We just got to noticin' that there was just a few too many of us young men — see, the men working in the company, we were young men. They were losin' too many guys. As we sat and ate and had our breaks, we just got to thinkin' that maybe there might be a little too much — too many of us guys just gettin' out of this world too young.

But who was counting the dead? No one. Throughout the 1960's, there had been no systematic mortality studies. The plastics industry did not initiate any. The law did not require any. And the federal government did not even have a staff capable of undertaking major occupational cancer studies.

Finally, when the National Institute for Occupational Safety and Health was created in 1971 as part of the Occupational Safety and Health Act, the federal government had, at last, an agency whose function was to perform epidemiologic field studies — to count the dead in order to benefit the living. NIOSH is organizationally situated within the Department of Health, Education and Welfare. From the beginning, it was understood that NIOSH would be a worker-oriented health protection agency. To its credit, the caliber of its work has been consistent with that purpose. With a staff of aggressive and conscientious scientists, there has never been any real problem with the quality of NIOSH's work. But there has always been a problem with the quantity. The Institute is starved for funds and for personnel. In the fiscal year 1975–76 NIOSH's entire budget for occupational cancer studies was $6.6 million — about eight cents a year for every American worker. To conduct a single study on the effects that a suspect carcinogen has had on the death rates of a defined population of workers costs $200,000 and occupies three people for two years. Since only forty-six full-time staff are devoted to these occupational cancer studies, it is obvious that only a handful of epidemiologic studies can be completed each year. As a result of this chronic underfunding, the backlog of both recognized and suspect carcinogens not yet fully examined by NIOSH grows ever larger: commercial talc, chloroprene, antimony, wood dust, lead, beryllium — there are scores of urgent studies left undone for lack of resources. Just to keep from being overwhelmed by this backlog, NIOSH needs at least another $10 million per year earmarked for occupational cancer.

Pumping additional resources into NIOSH is essential, but this alone is not enough. Something must be said about the primitive nature of occupational health record-keeping throughout the United States. The nation lacks even the most rudimentary occupational health record-keeping system. When NIOSH conducted its 1974 field survey at B. F. Goodrich, the study consisted essentially of matching employment records against death certificates. This rather straightforward task is made both complicated and costly by the fact that a worker leaving a job frequently moves to another county or state, making it difficult if not impossible to find out if he or she is alive or dead; and, if dead, to find the death certificate and the reported cause of death. The stories of this kind of epidemiologic detective work are frequently fascinating: medical sleuths spending endless hours poring through telephone books, contacting former neighbors, following up tips on the whereabouts of a long-lost employee. But amid the intriguing accounts of the chase, the larger lesson must not be lost: occupational cancer studies can take several years to complete precisely because the limited number of research personnel are bogged down in the horse-and-buggy age of occupational record-keeping in America.

It seems no exaggeration to suggest that if even a rudimentary occupational health record-keeping system had been available in 1960, the vinyl chloride cancer link could have been discovered five or ten years sooner, sparing hundreds and even thousands the agony of premature cancer deaths. What kind of a record-keeping system is needed? A good start would be a comprehensive national system that requires employers to annually record not only the name and social security number of the employee, but also the type of industry in which the worker is employed, the particular job, and the specific chemicals or physical agents that are being utilized on the job. This information could then be coded and stored in a government-owned computerized databank system. Then, as death certificates become available from county recorders across the country, these too would be entered into the databank and matched with appropriate employment records. Using a simple computer program, cancer deaths could then be routinely categorized according to industry, job function, and the specific substances to which employees were exposed. Cancer death trends could even be traced back to the individual companies involved. An early warning system: that's what a properly operated record-keeping system can offer. An early warning system that would enable government officials to spot suspicious cancer trends as they first emerged. An early warning system that might have saved Pete Gettelfinger's life, or at least given him more years before the onset of a fatal malignancy.

What other lessons are there to be learned from the vinyl chloride cancer pox? There is a lesson to be learned about the need for common sense cleanliness in industry. After the potent cancer-causing effects of vinyl chloride became evident in 1974, OSHA was prompted to promulgate new occupational health standards to limit worker exposure to vinyl chloride to as little as one part per million. Despite the industry's protests and dire predictions of the imminent collapse of the entire polyvinyl chloride industry, production today continues without major dislocations in terms of costs to the producers or to consumers. In the period after the vinyl chloride cancer link became public, in-plant exposure levels at major facilities were cut from 500 ppm — or more — to as little as 1 ppm. Interestingly, in the early 1960's, the Dow Chemical Company managed to cut vinyl chloride exposure levels to less than 50 ppm. Dow did this not because of any cancer fears — there were none at the time — but because of the sensible judgment that the needless inhalation of vinyl chloride gas, particularly in high doses, could not be good for human health and, indeed, was possibly very bad for human health. Dow's corporate colleagues, however, were doing little or nothing to cut vinyl chloride exposure levels. After all, no one had conclusively "proved" that the gas could be fatal to workers.

"Proof." What a perversion of science! In matters of cancer-causation, the demand for conclusive proof is invariably a carefully calculated stall. It is a way of invoking "science" as a basis for doing nothing to protect workers. Stripped of its pseudo-scientific veneer, the demand for conclusive proof is really a crude assertion that nothing will be done until the dead bodies are piled so high that there can no longer be any doubt. But the very purpose of science in the service of humanity is to cast doubt. To raise questions. To urge caution so that human life might be better protected. The shrill call for proof should be replaced by a common sense plea for prudence, care, and caution. If there is to be error in dealing with the unknown, let it be error on the side of health and life.

In practical terms, fundamental principles of sanitation must, at last, become legally binding upon those who profit financially from the industrial production of this nation. In homes and communities throughout the United States, citizens have long accepted the fact that dirt poses health hazards and that the control of dirt reduces those hazards. Cleanliness is generally recognized as a prudent preventive measure, protecting people not only against known health hazards, but against unknown health hazards too. The same principle should apply to industry. Industrial dirt, especially airborne chemical dirt, should be regarded as a potential health hazard in all instances. And the strict regulatory control of industrial dirt is the obvious means of reducing those hazards. It should not be necessary to marshal ironclad proof of a cancer epidemic or some other occupational calamity before common sense standards of industrial cleanliness are enforced as a matter of law throughout the United States.

Laws and regulations and enforcement. Government. Too much government, some say. Licensing and pretesting and record-keeping. There is too much government in our lives already, they say. But in matters of health in the plants and factories of America, just the opposite is true. It wasn't too much government that killed Pete Gettelfinger or Joe Fitman. On the contrary, these men died because there were no effective government controls reaching into their workplaces. There was no governmental presence to shield them from the unnecessary chemical abuses to which they were exposed. They were not victims of an overbearing government; they were victims of a brand of industrial anarchy — a production ethic that says anything goes until something goes wrong. It is an ethic that is utterly inappropriate in this perilous Chemical Age, an age in which an owner's unfettered corporate freedom may prove to be a worker's — and a nation's — cancer tragedy.

There is yet another lesson to emerge from the grief of the

vinyl chloride cancer pox. A bitter lesson of individual moral responsibility. Pete Gettelfinger posed the question and ventured an answer:

> And how long anybody knew that there was a cancer danger before I was told I had it? I don't know. But I suspect that someone knew up there for a while, somewhere in the industry, 'cause they had a product and they were sellin' it. You think about it. A year ago, angiosarcoma — the average man never heard of it. Too much has turned up too quick.

The vinyl chloride story broke in January 1974. But in mid-1973, there was a tightening of operations at B. F. Goodrich. The management was pressing workers to reduce vinyl chloride gas leaks and cut airborne exposure levels. Was this mopping up activity mere coincidence, unrelated to Maltoni's secret animal studies? It is possible, but it seems unlikely. Also in mid-1973, manufacturers of aerosol sprays, who had long used vinyl chloride gas as an aerosol propellant, began to switch from vinyl chloride to substitute propellants. Coincidence? Again, it is possible but unlikely. A more plausible explanation is that the word on Maltoni's cancerous rats was being quietly passed along to corporate executives at the highest tiers, and, from there, instructions were sent down to plant managers.

For more than three years, from late 1970 through early 1974, as the vinyl chloride cancer link moved from a working hypothesis to a proven fact, industry's representatives held the information in the strictest secrecy. Even amid the most serious suspicions of a major cancer risk to exposed workers, these representatives allowed hundreds of thousands of employees to go about their work as though there were nothing to fear. Also, during that period, the normal turnover of employees meant that tens of thousands of new workers, whose livers and brains and lungs had never before been subjected to the carcinogenic effect of vinyl chloride gas, had unwittingly been added to the population at risk. All of which raises the most disturbing question regarding industrial democracy: by what right do owners and managers withhold information — literally life-and-death information — from the men and women they employ?

Cancer is far too serious a disease to permit any misunderstanding on the issue of individual moral and legal responsibility. Recognizing the heightened cancer hazards in a chemicalized society, the responsibility of corporate officers must, by legislation, be understood to include much more than the single-minded notion of maximizing profit. Federal law should impose upon corporate officials the obligation to fully disclose — not just to government agencies but also to employees and employee representatives — all information that even hints at a possible cancer risk to exposed workers. The law should make clear that a knowing violation would constitute a felony, punishable by imprisonment. Cancer is a disease of such an insidious nature — its onset generally unknown to its victim, its effect so frequently lethal — that the failure to disclose information concerning an industrial cancer hazard should be regarded as the equivalent of a felonious assault. And when there are dead victims as a result of a willful nondisclosure, the crime should be regarded as homicide. Industrial homicide. For here, as with any other kind of homicide, what is involved is willful conduct that results in the taking of another person's life.

On the issue of moral responsibility for the cancer deaths of others, Rita Gettelfinger still holds to her point of view:

> But . . . you have to go back to the old theory that every man has been appointed one day to answer. And if he knew and didn't do anything about it, he's going to have to answer.

Surely, if there is "one day to answer," it is not unreasonable to make those who have perpetrated such crimes answer twice — the first time here on earth, before a jury of peers.

Part III

Chapter 5.

Dr. Peter Capurro

IT WOULD BE DIFFICULT to imagine a more picturesque landscape. Little Elk Valley is located in the northeast corner of Maryland, several miles removed from the closest town. It is indeed a little valley — no more than three square miles and populated by about 120 people.* Coming up the narrow winding road from the south, the valley's natural beauty is quickly evident. A small stream, called Little Elk Creek, flows from north to south through occasional meadows. Bridges are laid across the creek every few hundred yards. And the trees — dogwood, maple, elm — there are trees everywhere in the valley. Near the creek. On the hillsides. In spring and summer, wildflowers of all colors are in bloom. But in the fall, it is the trees that provide the color.

In the summer of 1967, Dr. Peter Capurro, a pathologist, first came to Little Elk Valley. He was looking for a place to live for himself and his family. He recalled later that when he saw the valley, he felt he had discovered "a little Shangri-la." As luck would have it, among the few dozen dwellings in the valley, there was a house for sale. It was an impressive brick structure, just the right size and in good condition. Adjacent to the house was a sizeable pond, a habitat for wild ducks. A path lined with azaleas, geraniums, and tulips separated the house and the pond. Thinking back, the doctor says, "It seemed a dream world." He quickly bought the house. Within weeks the Capurros moved in — the doctor, his wife, Dorothy, and their two children, Claudia, then seven years old, and Christopher, five.

---

*Little Elk Valley actually encompasses a somewhat larger area and population. The smaller community, described in the narrative, is the geographically distinct southern end of the valley.

The first weekend they were at the house, Dr. Capurro happened to be in the kitchen when he noticed a peculiar odor. At first it smelled like manure. Then at times the odor seemed sweet-smelling. He stepped outside and walked around the house, but was unable to locate the source of the foul smell. Finally, he called a neighbor, who told him that the odors came from the nearby Galaxy Chemical Company. Although it was ten o'clock in the evening, Capurro looked up Galaxy in the telephone book and dialed the number. When a worker answered, the doctor wasted no time with niceties. He asked straight out if they were dumping chemicals in Little Elk Creek. The worker at the other end answered, "Yes." Then he asked if the chemicals were harmful to people. Again, "Yes." Do they damage the lungs? The worker didn't know.

The next day, Dr. Capurro called the county commissioner to complain. Then he called Galaxy's president, Mr. Paul J. Mraz. When he got Mraz on the phone, the doctor told him he smelled odors around the house that seemed to be chemical solvents — perhaps a mixture of benzene, toluene, and xylene. Because of an unfortunate incident, Capurro was familiar with chemical solvents. Once before, when working in a hospital, he had been exposed to solvents through a faulty ventilation system. The experience had left him with a temporarily paralyzed left side and a rapidly fluctuating blood pressure. Ironically, the Capurros had come to Maryland to recover — to get away from chemical hazards. Responding to Capurro's concern, Mraz was pleasant but noncommittal about the matter. Nevertheless, he agreed to visit Dr. Capurro at his home to talk things over. When he arrived, Mraz explained that Galaxy was handling chemicals, but he denied that any significant odors were emitted. The doctor asked him if he had any carbon tetrachloride at the plant. Mraz denied it. The doctor said he felt certain that Galaxy was working with benzene, toluene, and xylene — he knew what they smelled like. Mraz held firm in his denial, provoking Dr. Capurro to escalate the encounter one notch. Capurro asserted that he would prove the presence of solvents in the air. Mraz asked him how, and the doctor replied, "With a gas chromatograph — to analyze air samples." At this point, Mraz abandoned his pleasant disposition, telling the doctor that he couldn't prove anything. Then, thoroughly exasperated at the bluntness of the Italian-born physician, Mraz added, "You can't even speak English."

Paul Mraz badly misjudged his adversary. Dr. Capurro speaks an uneven, heavily accented English. In appearance, he is rather ordinary. He has a gentle-looking face, framed by heavy glasses. He is balding and slightly paunchy. At fifty-one years of age, he has the look of a man well suited to a sedentary, middle-age lifestyle. But in fact, his appearance tends to mask a most unusual personality — a man of enormous energy, talent, and tenacity. Dr. Pietro Capurro was born in Genoa, Italy, in 1925. He graduated from the University of Genoa Medical School in 1951. During the Second World War, he fought in the Italian Underground against the Nazis. In 1953, he came to the United States as a resident in pathology at Kings County Hospital in Brooklyn, New York. A few years later, he did further work in pathology at the Mount Sinai Hospital in Cleveland, Ohio. There, he studied under Dr. Harry Goldblatt, a distinguished researcher responsible for important breakthroughs in the treatment of kidney disease, In the mid-1950's, Goldblatt provided Capurro with the opportunity to engage in cancer research involving chemical carcinogenesis in small animals. During the late 1950's and 1960's, Dr. Capurro taught pathology to medical students. He also directed a hospital laboratory in Alton, Illinois. Finally, in 1966, he took a position as Director of Laboratories at Union Hospital in Cecil County, Maryland, only seven miles from the home he later purchased in Little Elk Valley.

Dr. Capurro became an American citizen on Saint Valentine's Day in 1962. In the years since, he has shown that he is not only a skilled physician, but a man who, by instinct and experience, has developed a special sense of citizenship, an uncommon willingness to stand up against irresponsible authority whether it is exercised by corporate officers or public officials. This trait would soon become evident as the Little Elk Valley controversy got underway.

True to his word, Dr. Capurro set out to prove that the Galaxy Chemical Company was polluting the water and air of the Little Elk Valley with dangerous chemicals. Until his meeting with Mraz, the doctor hadn't even known of Galaxy's existence. He soon learned that the plant was not only nearby; it was wedged in at the north end of Little Elk Valley, just a mile from his home.

Galaxy is a small outfit employing perhaps two dozen workers. The plant is an old brick building with a tall chimney. It used to be a paper mill until it was gutted by fire in 1954. Seven years later, in 1961, Galaxy bought the plant and converted it for reclaiming solvents from discarded chemicals. By the truckload, chemical wastes are transported to Galaxy from a number of East Coast industrial plants and then distilled to recover certain chemicals for resale. After his initial inspection of the plant, Dr. Capurro wrote down his impressions.

Only one worker was present at the plant. The plant was a stinking mess. At the rear of the plant two ponds are present. One black containing black material and one containing a yellowish watery fluid. These ponds emit a very acrid odor. On the grounds of the plant deep puddles of chemicals are present. Small streams of chemicals can be seen making their way toward the creek. The underground is combed with pipes. And an opening of pipes is present in the front of the plant. Several openings can be seen on the bank of the creek.

After this first survey, Capurro soon began to gather evidence with the gas chromatograph, an expensive machine that measures solvent vapors and other chemicals present in a small sample of air or water. At first he took daytime air samples. Then he realized that the chemical dumping was an around-the-clock matter, with perhaps the heaviest discharges taking place in the early morning hours. And, so, on repeated occasions, he went out at night to gather evidence. Typically, after going to sleep in the evening, he would awaken at one or two o'clock in the morning, feeling pain in his stomach and chest because of his sensitivity to solvents. Like a biological alarm clock, this was his signal that chemicals were heavy in the air. His equipment in hand, Dr. Capurro wandered out, taking air and water samples in special syringes and injecting them into two separate gas chromatographs.

I would take a reading and would find there was never one chemical in the air. At least two. Often six or seven. Up to fifteen at one time. I was going out night, day. Two o'clock, three o'clock at night. Sunday, Saturday. Two o'clock at night there were very high readings. I went down and through the creek and up on the hills. One night I went to a lagoon to test it and fell with one leg in the black lagoon. Right into the chemicals. I lost all the hair on my leg! I had to throw away my suit and shoes and stockings. But in the pond I found toluene and other chemicals. This was the first time I knew that toluene was present for certain at the plant, although I had already found toluene in the air near my house.

Toluene. One of many industrial solvents. Solvents are chemicals that dissolve things, such as grease and oil, paint and lacquer. But solvents also dissolve in the human body, causing temporary or permanent damage. The damage frequently produces quick symptoms: headaches, nausea, dizziness, lethargy, difficulty in breathing. Some of the solvents lead to biologic damage that is without apparent symptoms. Like blood changes. And damage to cells that ultimately may lead to cancer.

Soon, Dr. Capurro was able to provide a fairly comprehensive list of the chemical solvents present in the valley's air and water. In addition to toluene, he found benzene, carbon tetrachloride and methyl ethyl ketone — all toxic substances, some suspected or confirmed cancer-causing agents. Then, in an important new dimension to his study, he took blood samples from many of the valley's residents and found these same chemical agents present at abnormally high levels. Ever the scientist, he began to notice and learn about the movement of chemicals. Contrary to what might be expected, the airborne chemicals did not disperse evenly throughout the valley the way water might fill a lake. The chemicals had a tendency to move along certain pathways —

down along the banks of the Little Elk Creek, up a road, through a ravine. These pathways seemed to be formed by the wind and the local topography. On one side of the road, near a ravine, the chemicals might be heavily concentrated. Yet, on the other side of the road, readings might show only a small concentration. The doctor also discovered that chemicals might move along in an airborne cluster, then bump into a hill or a group of trees and be bounced along a new pathway. His study was more than just an academic exercise. As chief pathologist at the nearby Union Hospital, he soon encountered the most disturbing clinical findings.

About '68, '69, I think about people from the valley that were getting sick — fatigue, nausea, headaches. I diagnosed several cases of pancreatitis [inflammation of the pancreas] *— several at the same time — when there had been high levels of solvents in the air. Then, a little later, I start to think about cancer. I noticed that there was some increased incidence of lymphomas because Mrs. Nelson* died of lymphoma and Mr. Thompson died of lymphoma. Then I had a patient that I did an autopsy on, Mr. Rogers, who died of lymphoma. So three lymphomas. Then my neighbor Benson developed leukemia.*

It was about 1969 that I started looking at the possibility of increased incidence of tumors. Then, there was another man, a man who worked at the plant. His name was Weaver, Michael Weaver. He was twenty-one years old when I diagnosed him for carcinoma of the pancreas. He went down, on my suggestion, to the University of Maryland where they confirmed the diagnosis, I've been told. He died a few months later in our hospital. He was an extremely nice fellow. He worked for six months at the plant when he started to get sick. He asked me, "Do you think the chemicals caused the disease?" At that time it was still early, and I said, "I don't know. I don't know enough to give you an answer." Now, Mr. Mraz and the doctor who was taking care of him — they said he was sick before working for the plant. He told me it was not true. Now, the doctor that was taking care of him — he was a very good friend of Mraz. So, I

---

*The actual names of patients have been changed to respect requirements of confidentiality.

*don't know what was true. I have a tendency to believe the patients, not
the doctor or Mraz.*

*Weaver married just before he died. He wanted to get married before
he died. He was a very wonderful fellow. A very nice person. I had a very
strong feeling for him and also for Mr. Rogers. Rogers was a very nice
person. Very quiet. He came to us to help him three days before he died.
He said he wanted to fight the plant. He said, "I feel so sick from the
smell." Rogers wasn't bitter. He was passive at the end. Quiet. When I
saw people die I would get more determined to fight. When the people
would die, I would get more stubborn.*

*Out of nine cancers from the valley, I diagnosed five. This was too
much. I would think I diagnose too much from this area in comparison to
the rest of the county. So I really started to look in 1973, together with
Mr. [Carl] York of the Maryland State Health Department [Bureau of
Air Quality Control]. I found there was increased incidence. For some,
I had their name. York, he knew some who died of malignancies. I took
the data, put it all together, and made a short report for the State Health
Department. Actually, we made it together, York and me. For those living
there more than five years, the death rate from cancer was about five
times higher than it should have been.*

A cancer death rate "about five times higher than it should
have been." But even more alarming were the breakdowns on
the kinds of cancer people were dying from in the Little Elk Valley. Over a seven-year period, four had died of lymphomas —
cancer of the lymph-forming tissues. This is more than sixty
times the expected death rate from malignant lymphomas. The
chance that so many lymphomas would randomly occur in a
population of 120 people is less than one in 100,000. Another
two residents suffered from pancreatic tumors. The probability
of observing two tumors of the pancreas in a population that
small is six in 1000. Coupled with these startling statistics was the
fact that these two types of cancer — lymphomas and tumors of
the pancreas — are increasingly common among chemists. In
fact, at almost the precise time that Dr. Capurro was puzzling
over the cancer riddle of Little Elk Valley, a National Cancer In-
situte study was underway among members of the American

Chemical Society, who were dying from cancer at a rate nearly 25 percent higher than that of other professional groups. And almost half of the excess deaths among the chemists were due to malignancies of the lymph glands or the pancreas.

Dr. Capurro was a worried man. His clinical and statistical surveys pointed to an extraordinary cancer risk to valley residents, including his own family. These findings, when published, were also creating another kind of health hazard for the doctor and his family. Capurro's mailbox was damaged or destroyed seven times. Stinking chemicals were thrown at his house. His automobile tires were slashed. Finally, in May 1972 he sold his house and moved his family out of the valley. But he did not quit. He continued to document the alarming excess of cancer deaths among the valley's 120 residents. Beyond this, he began to develop a sophisticated hypothesis about the cancer epidemic in Little Elk Valley. Knowing as he did that Galaxy was dumping benzene, carbon tetrachloride, and other suspected cancer-causing chemicals, and that the chemicals tended to move along certain pathways, he made house-by-house readings of chemical concentrations. He found generally that those struck down by cancer had had the misfortune of living in houses situated in a chemical pathway. While he cautiously avoided any public charges, he hypothesized that Galaxy was the cause of the elevated incidence of cancer, and that within the valley the risks were unevenly distributed among the residents, depending upon where they were located in relation to the chemical pathways that he had charted.

Capurro spent endless hours working on the problem — amassing data, studying topographical maps, checking and rechecking wind patterns. But as he grew closer to a detailed explanation of the cancer tragedy of Little Elk Valley, he realized that his painstaking work was largely ignored by those who should value it most — the government officials charged with protecting the public's health.

I always furnished every data I got immediately to the State Department of Health. I was calling them, saying what I was finding — everything. They were ignoring it. They would say, "Maybe." Then they would say, "How can you prove it? Can you give your papers to us so we can look?" If I give my papers, they say, "We don't understand what it means. We don't understand. We don't know how to read it." So it was ridiculous. All this for them — for the State of Maryland — is a comedy. It is incredible. Oh, I think it is terrible. Even the Environmental Protection Agency . . .

I thought at the beginning I could believe them, you know. When we moved there I talked to them — the government officials. I was calling them nights. I even call up the White House. I talked with two associates of Mr. Nixon. I think one of them was John Dean. He send me a lot of paper showing how much Nixon does to control pollution. Anybody I could, I contacted because it was so incredible that this could happen — that it would be allowed to happen. I said there must be somebody in this country that cares. There wasn't. There isn't. Maybe except the newspapers, I guess. I started with the county. Then I started at the state level. We sent telegrams to Agnew [then Governor of Maryland]. *We wrote to Agnew. He gave it to the health department. We wrote to this new governor, too — Mandel. I talk with everybody at the health department. With universities. I wrote lawyers. I wrote to senators. Congressmen. I wrote to Muskie. He never answered.*

Refusing to be overlooked, the doctor joined in efforts to publicize what was going on in Little Elk Valley.

The person who publicized it here was not me really. It was Dr. Kailin.* She came. She was hired by the State Health Department to check the health problem. They were decided there was no pollution — the State Health Department. For them it was all my invention. There was no chemicals in the air. Things were perfectly clean there. But they said we'll do another thing. We send Dr. Kailin to check it to see if there is any health problem. And Dr. Kailin came and said, yes, there is a health problem. But, then, to them Dr. Kailin became a "nut," "no good," because she agreed with me. They knew her. They hire her. But she agrees with me so they said she was a nut.

What Kailin did, she knew some people at the Sentinel, *and she told the story to the reporter from the* Sentinel. *So they wrote an article —*

---

*Dr. Eloise Kailin is a specialist in allergies and environmental medicine.

front page of the Sentinel. *This was picked up by the* Washington Post *and they wrote some two or three articles about Galaxy. The* Washington Post *was picked up by the* National Observer — *front page. And then it was picked up by television. At the beginning publicity was not my doing . . . but I found myself in the middle of it . . . So it was Kailin; she got so mad at the State Health Department that she went to the newspapers. Then the newspapers looked for me. They felt I was the one to talk to.*

When the *Washington Post* interviewed Capurro for a front page article about Little Elk Valley in August 1974, he managed to collect his syntax and summarize the meaning of the evidence he had gathered. "I can't say that the deaths in the valley from cancer were the result of specific exposure to chemical fumes. But there have been a lot of chemicals in that valley's air and water and the blood of those people we tested, and some of those chemicals cause cancer. And we know there are a lot more malignancies there than you would expect . . . If you're in a room where everyone is scratched and there's a lion in there, too, then you've got to suspect the lion."

The *Post* article included statements by some of the valley's residents. The most colorful of the locals was Olive Feehly, an elderly lady who ran a small general store with her husband, George. The store was less than 200 yards west of the plant. Mrs. Feehly counted off on her fingers the names of her neighbors who had died recently. "This used to be a place where people died of old age and you'd go years without a funeral sometimes. Good Lord, nowadays I spend more time in the funeral parlor than I do in my own home."

After the *Washington Post* article appeared, the CBS Evening News spotlighted the Little Elk Valley cancer episode in a five-minute news segment.

I think publicity — it's the only pressure you can get on the congressmen and senators because they don't want to think about it. Even the local level. Let's put it this way: I wrote to tell some senators and congressmen. They . . . no answer. I told on the television that I wrote to these people and have not received an answer — the following day they were all on the telephone from their offices. If you go on the television and tell that they don't answer, it doesn't sound good!

Even in the face of all this — the adverse publicity, the seemingly obvious connection between Galaxy's dumping of chemical carcinogens and the five-fold increase in cancer deaths among valley residents — the state public health officials remained unmoved. Rather than test Dr. Capurro's hypothesis — correlating the cancer epidemic to the flow of chemical carcinogens through the Little Elk Valley — the State Department of Health refused to even acknowledge that there have been excess cancer deaths in the valley. They argued, instead, that the doctor should use a larger sample, one that included hundreds of more people outside the immediate confines of the valley. But, of course, this is directly contrary to Capurro's hypothesis that this particular cancer epidemic is a local one because of the proximity of the valley's 120 residents to Galaxy and its resultant carcinogenic pathways.

More than anything else, it is this transparent attempt to cover up evidence of a localized cancer epidemic that infuriates the doctor.

The state agencies — a waste of money. They are worthless! Not only worthless, but they are also so basically directed to lying. Incredible. They make it up in lying what they don't do in action. It's unbelievable.

In a more philosophical vein, he recalls the lessons taught by the Norwegian playwright, Henrik Ibsen. In 1882, Ibsen wrote his classic play *Enemy of the People,* about a small-town physician who discovers that the town's mineral baths — its main tourist attraction — have become contaminated. He urges that the baths be shut down at once. Instead of being regarded as a benefactor of public health, the doctor is scorned — by businessmen, by the town's political leaders, and by its public health officials. They all have a stake in disbelieving the bad news. And, when the doctor confronts them with strident demands to protect the health of unsuspecting tourists, they at first dismiss his claims; then they attack his integrity; and, finally, they brand him an outcast. An enemy of the people. Dr. Capurro believes the same kinds of institutional forces are at work in the Little Elk Valley cancer controversy.

How does he deal with it all? There is anger. But it is anger that is channeled so that it seems to reinforce his determination rather than erode it. And beyond the anger, there is a strain of optimism suggesting that Capurro is convinced that the truth will ultimately prevail; that his hypothesis will be accepted and acted upon by those in positions of authority. In the meantime, he patiently explains the evidence to those who seek him out in search of a story. If asked, he will trek to the Little Elk Valley to point out the particulars of the problem.

The tour includes impromptu visits with valley residents. On one of these visits in November 1974, he stopped to see Olive Feehly at her store in order to have her talk with a couple of reporters. She wouldn't talk to the reporters. She said she felt sick and not at all up to giving an interview. Outside the store, Capurro explained to the reporters that she was too ill to talk, adding, "She is sick too much. I think it is cancer of the pancreas."

In addition to whatever publicity he can give the issue, Dr. Capurro has written several scientific papers about Little Elk Valley. They constitute an effort to interest his colleagues not only in this particular cancer epidemic, but also in the larger issue of chemical pollution and its devastating consequences to health. The doctor has the qualities of a teacher as well as a crusader.

The biggest problem to understand is the movement of chemicals in the air. For instance, in a city it would channel along the road. It would be very interesting to study what happened on the prevailing wind side of the road. Take Los Angeles — a plant next to a freeway. A chemical from a plant along the freeway — it would channel along the freeway. That would be an enormous place of chemical movement. And it would be nice to compare the symptoms and diseases in the houses on one side of the road compared to the other. A river — you'll have the same thing — a chemical channel. A chemical from a plant four, five miles away. It goes up, comes down. Follows the river. In Switzerland. a doctor said that he found increased malignancies along roads.

I think people that are exposed to chemicals in one way — in their own home or from a plant nearby — they may get irritable. Fatigue. Headaches. They go to the doctor and the doctor will tell them, "Oh, we don't find what you have." Or, "It's all in your head." Or, "You need a tranquilizer." Or, "You need to be pepped up on some pill." So we have a lot of people taking pills and not being treated for what they have. So this I feel should be a new phase of medicine. The medical schools should recognize it. They should offer a new field, like they offered microbiology years ago. And they should start to analyze the problem that exists. I don't think that most of the medical schools are ready today. You see, we cannot continue to think that only bacteria are what affect the human. Many more things besides bacteria affect the human body. A hundred years ago they didn't want to accept the idea of bacteria. Now we have to start thinking in terms of new ideas again — but this time using the gas chromatograph to measure chemical exposures.

And what does Capurro feel about Galaxy's president, Mr. Mraz, and those who have frustrated his efforts to protect the handful of citizens who inhabit the star-crossed Little Elk Valley?

You see, I don't blame Mraz. He has to make a living. I blame the State Health Department. Any individual big or small — especially small — will try to get away with what they can get away. And the people who should control them are the State Health Department. Now, if this small industry cannot solve the problem by themselves, then the State Health Department or the federal government ought to come in and do something helpful. They should give money, cheap loans, money at really low interest to make conditions proper for the plant to work or even to place it somewhere else where it's more proper for the plant to work. The state is wasting more money doing all what it's doing to shut me up than if they would come in and solve the problem.

I look at it this way. I did the best I could with what I knew. I didn't lie. I did the work I could. Within my limits I went all the way. I didn't save my money. If I needed money, I would spend it. I did not avoid any work for myself. I tell the things like they are. Like I see it.

I am peaceful about all this . . . Dr. Goldblatt — he is a wonderful man — *he taught me. He told me, "Say the truth and it doesn't matter what happens to you afterward." So I am saying the truth. I say I can make mistakes, but they will not be dishonest mistakes. Anybody who does something can possibly make a mistake. I say to them, "Please, help me. I'm ready to work with you. I'm ready to work with Mraz." I said to Mraz, "I'm ready to give to you my gas chromatograph to help you if you really want to correct the plant."*

I'm not after shutting down Mraz. I don't hate Mraz. I'm disgusted with the place, but I am not afraid. I accept that it can be very dangerous for me, you know. The state can do anything. The only protection I have is newspapers. The only protection I have may be the news media in a free society. Mraz, you see — I don't talk well about him, but I don't feel any hostility. The others — the health officials — I feel it.

Chapter 6.

Beyond the Factory Gates

IN RECENT MONTHS, there have been important developments in Little Elk Valley. Galaxy Chemical Company, always a marginal operation, found its creditors foreclosing on existing loans in November 1975. For a brief time, it appeared that the firm might go out of business. In satisfying its creditors, about half of Galaxy's equipment was sold off. But according to Paul Mraz, the remaining equipment would be used in a new commercial process: refining antifreeze. Presumably no longer heavily involved in reclaiming solvents, the company has been given a new lease on life. As for the citizens who populate the valley, they have not been so fortunate. Olive Feehly, the sixty-nine-year-old proprietor of the small general store, died in March 1975. The cause of death was, as Dr. Capurro had believed, cancer of the pancreas. Another cancer coincidence? Or a cancer pox? Even before Olive Feehly's death, the evidence was reaching irrefutable proportions. Then, fifteen months after Olive died, her husband, George, died from lymphoma, the valley's fifth case of lymphoma.

The State of Maryland, always the dutiful disbeliever, was finally moved to conduct a study that it completed in late 1975. The most crucial statistic: valley residents (before the fifth case of lymphoma had been diagnosed) are dying from lymphatic cancer at a rate thirty times greater than normal. Because of the irreversible biologic damage already incurred by the living, the number and rate of cancer fatalities are sure to increase still further. All the classic characteristics are there: carcinogenic exposures, the long latency period — frequently ten years or more — and then the excessive cancer deaths. This improbable place, Little Elk Valley, Maryland, is the site of a cancer epidemic — the epidemic in slow motion.

And the governmental response? It remains meager. For five years, the federal Environmental Protection Agency, with offices less than 100 miles away in Washington, D.C., demonstrated only passing interest in the Little Elk Valley situation. Finally, in the spring of 1976, the EPA stationed a trailer in the valley to record air samples. But with Galaxy assertedly phasing out of the solvent business, the EPA testing can now do little to explain the nature and extent of what went on before. In the past, NIOSH, which is reponsible for surveying worker health, indicated some interest in the valley's cancer problem, but backed off for lack of available resources. In the bureaucratese of one federal official: "We have other priorities taking our manpower and time. We feel some aspects of the valley's situation are interesting, though, and we may consider some kind of contractual study for a full evaluation some time in the future." Translation: in sheer numbers — the number of people involved and the number of human lives at stake — Little Elk Valley is a pee-wee operation. There are bigger concerns that have first call on the limited resources of federal government agencies.

What is lost in this response is a creative understanding of the significance of the Little Elk Valley controversy. If a scientist were to set out to design a model to test the cancer-causing effects of industrial carcinogens upon a limited, locally exposed population, he or she would be hard pressed to find a better model than that which has existed in the Little Elk Valley. The valley's geography effectively gives the area a nearly perfect test tube quality. It is geographically isolated. Its resident population is limited. And there has been but one source of intense chemical pollution — the Galaxy Chemical Company. Like any other test tube model, its real importance lies in what it tells us about the world beyond the test tube. The Little Elk Valley tragedy tells us a great deal.

It tells us most if we ask the question: What if the Galaxy Chemical Company had never located in Little Elk Valley but had located instead in a neighborhood in Wilmington, Delaware, for instance? Of course, a likely consequence would have been that the residents of Little Elk Valley, Maryland, would have been spared the cancer calamity that has befallen them. But what of the residents of Wilmington, Delaware, who lived in the homes and apartments surrounding the plant? They, rather than the Little Elk Valley residents, would have incurred the repeated carcinogenic insults that apparently lead to an excessive cancer rate. But who would have known? Who would have made the discovery? Probably no one. The tangle of urban life in Wilmington is so complex that the variables can never be satisfactorily sorted out. To begin with, there are many more people, and they move in and out by the thousands each year. They receive medical attention — and cancer diagnoses — from many different physicians, none of whom would be likely to see enough pieces to understand the whole puzzle. Six or seven excess cancer deaths in the Little Elk Valley, observed by one physician, is a striking occurrence. But in Wilmington, Delaware, six or seven excess cancer deaths spread over several years — or even sixty or seventy excess cancer deaths spread over several years — would probably go unnoticed. The population base is simply too large.

So much for hypothetical situations. The fact is that across the United States hundreds upon hundreds of Galaxy-type operations are running daily. In Wilmington, the so-called Chemical Capital of the World, in Chicago, in St. Louis, in New York, in Birmingham. If there is any difference at all, it is only one of scale. For in Wilmington and elsewhere, the plants that do essentially the same kind of work — involving the massive use of chemical solvents — are perhaps fifty or 100 times the size of the Galaxy Chemical Company. What is happening in Little Elk Valley, Maryland, *is* happening in scores of industrial centers throughout America. However, outside the test tube of Little Elk Valley, the tragedy is more diffuse. It is spread over a much larger population. And, so, it is less obvious.

This is not a case of fanciful theorizing. Clinical and statistical data exist, confirming that the cancer pox is spreading beyond the occupational setting. Even at this early point, the community clinical evidence against vinyl chloride is emerging. Victims of angiosarcoma of the liver have been reported among citizens who never worked with vinyl chloride but who have lived for some time near a vinyl chloride plant. The Connecticut Tumor Registry reported two recent cases of angiosarcoma among residents of the Bridgeport-Stratford area. Neither of the victims had a history of occupational exposures. One resident had lived his entire life within two miles of an important industrial source of vinyl chloride; the other, an elderly housewife, had lived within one-half mile of a vinyl products plant. Angiosarcoma of the liver is so rare that this southwestern sector of Connecticut should generate less than one case in ten years. But, in fact, the Connecticut Tumor Registry reveals five local cases in the past ten years, four of them occurring in 1972 and 1973. Coincidence? Or cancer pox? In 1974, United States plastics producers discharged more than *200 million pounds* of vinyl chloride into the air — into the unseen chemical pathways like those Dr. Capurro charted in the Little Elk Valley.

Asbestos offers similar evidence. Mesothelioma — the tumor that attacks the lining of the lungs or abdominal cavity — seems to be almost exclusively the product of exposure to inhaled asbestos fibers. In addition to asbestos workers struck down by the malignancy, doctors report numerous "neighborhood cases" of the disease. One case involved a woman who died from mesothelioma at the age of forty-four. When she was a child, her father had worked the late shift at the Union Asbestos and Rubber Company in Paterson, New Jersey, and each evening she took him a hot meal, waiting outside the plant until he picked it up. Another case involved a woman who, before she died, recalled her countless hours of childhood play in a local asbestos dump.

Dr. Muriel L. Newhouse, of the Department of Occupational Health at the London School of Hygiene and Tropical Medicine, recently contributed important evidence concerning community hazards from asbestos exposure. Dr. Newhouse investigated seventy-six cases of mesothelioma that had been confirmed by autopsy or biopsy. To no one's surprise, thirty-one of the seventy-six patients had worked with asbestos. Of the remaining forty-five who had never worked with asbestos, Dr. Newhouse learned that eleven of these cancer victims had lived within one-half mile of an asbestos factory.

Beyond the clinical cases, there are the mounting statistical data illustrating the fact that the occupational cancer epidemic is spreading into the general community. A study of Los Angeles County cancer rates recently reported a markedly higher incidence of lung cancer among residents in the heavily industrialized south-central area. The study attributed the excess lung cancers to particularly high levels of benzo(a)pyrene, a carcinogen that is probably formed of effluents from the petroleum and chemical industries concentrated in the area. Years earlier, a similar study on Staten Island, New York, disclosed that unusually high lung cancer rates in certain parts of the island seemed to be related to local wind conditions and the resulting exposure to airborne industrial carcinogens originating at nearby oil refineries.

More statistical evidence: in 1975, the National Cancer Institute published an *Atlas of Cancer Mortality for U.S. Counties: 1950–1969* showing the county-by-county variations in cancer death rates across the United States for sixteen common anatomic sites of the disease. The *Atlas* is an intriguing 103-page document that includes sixty-six separate color-coded maps of the United States. Each map is a mosaic of bright colors painted into oddly shaped little areas corresponding to county boundaries or state economic areas. Some areas are colored red. Others blue. Still others are green or yellow. The irony is inescapable: these maps, so lively and colorful, represent the geography of gray, malignant death. But more than irony is present here. The *Atlas* provides important clues to the factors contributing to cancer causation in industrialized American communities. For example, on the color-coded map depicting the geography of lung cancer, splotches of yellow, orange, and red — the colors indicating above-average lung cancer death rates — appear in counties where a significant percentage of the work force is engaged in smelting and refining copper, lead, and zinc ores. Inorganic arsenic, a known carcinogen, is an airborne by-product of the smelting of these ores. But this is not simply one further example of occupationally induced cancer; the data demonstrate above-average lung cancer rates for females as well as males in these counties. The meaning of this seems clear: the occupational cancer risk from arsenic, once limited to the men working with the substance, is now threatening whole communities.

Communties like Kellogg, Idaho. Idaho. Fresh air and open spaces and blue skies — some of the alluring qualities of the American Northwest. But in Kellogg, Idaho, where the Bunker Hill Company operates a huge lead smelter, the skies have become the carcinogenic pathways carrying the gray, metalloid crystals of arsenic into the lives and lungs of the Kellogg citizenry. In Shoshone County, where Kellogg is located, the lung cancer mortality rate for white males was 61 percent greater than the statewide lung cancer rate. And for white females, it was 80 percent greater than the statewide rate. While children are too young to manifest and succumb to lung cancer, their lungs and lymphatic systems, their guts, and their skins absorb the arsenic. Their cell systems suffer the silent violence of carcinogenic bombardment as they grow from infants, to toddlers, to adolescents, to adults.

But atmospheric pathways are not the only carriers of carcinogens. There are human pathways, too. In Kellogg, at the end of a long day, workers trek home from the plant. There, they shed their arsenic-covered clothes, to be handled, shaken, and washed — turning the household into a repository for a "take-home" carcinogen. This is not a trifling occurrence. In the case of asbestos, another notorious take-home carcinogen, a recent study using x-rays shows that more than 35 percent of the people who had lived in the same house with an asbestos worker developed lung abnormalities characteristic of occupational asbestos exposure.

Asbestos and arsenic are visible, tangible substances. But the take-home danger can apply to gases, too. Like vinyl chloride. Rita Gettelfinger remembers:

When Ray would come home, his clothes smelled from the various [substances he made from the vinyl chloride gas]. Like the acrylates. If he would come in in the winter time, his shoes, his coat — I mean he'd just have to almost put them outside. Or he'd come in on the four-to-twelve shift and I'd get up the next morning and I'd say, "Huh, you've been workin' in acrylates," 'cause I mean I could smell 'em on the other side of the room.

Carcinogenic pathways are abundant. In addition to human and atmospheric pathways, local and regional waterways have become the liquid pathways that carry industrial carcinogens into the general community. In November 1974, Dr. Robert Harris of the Environmental Defense Fund released the results of a major study that sought to explain the disturbingly high rate of cancer deaths in New Orleans, Louisiana. The conclusion was that the excessive deaths were primarily the result of cancers of the digestive and excretory organs. And these cancers, in turn, could be linked to the carcinogen-laden drinking water obtained from the Mississippi River.

The drinking water! How did it happen? Long before the Ojibway Indians named it Missi Sipi — the Great River — the Mississippi River moved along its meandering 4000-mile course, essentially free of cancer-causing substances as it flowed from the northern snowfields through the center of what is now the United States, draining over 40 percent of this land mass, and emptying into the Gulf of Mexico. But in the past century, the Mississippi River, like the Ohio River, the Hudson River, and the Little Elk Creek — like thousands of American waterways great and small — has become an industrial sewer. A convenient chemical dump for countless industries. And a receptacle for scores of toxic substances, many of them known cancer-causing agents. In January 1976, the General Electric Company acknowledged that it was dumping polychlorinated biphenyls (PCB's) — a liver carcinogen — into the Hudson River. According to GE, the dumping was taking place under a permit granted by the EPA, even though the agency had entered into an international agreement in 1973 to curb further environmental contamination with this potent carcinogen.

PCB's provide but one more addition to the lengthening list of waterborne carcinogens. America's rivers now carry cancer-causing petroleum wastes — fuel oils, lubricating oils, and cutting oils. They carry coal tar, pitch, creosote, and anthracene oil — all confirmed carcinogens. They carry carcinogens from dye and rubber industries — beta-Naphthylamine, benzidine, and 4-Aminodiphenyl. And on top of this burden there is a cruel chemical irony: chlorine, the agent historically used in treatment plants to kill waterborne bacteria, may react with certain industrial pollutants to actually produce new cancer-causing compounds. For example, chlorine reacts with acetone to become chloroform, a carcinogen that can be found in significant quantities in an ordinary glass of drinking water. And in the food prepared with water. And in the steamy mist that accompanies a hot shower.

There are those who scoff at such matters, taking refuge in the fantasy that because the waterborne carcinogen levels are low-dose, they, therefore, must fall within some mythical "margin of safety." What is overlooked here is the cumulative nature of the cancerization process. For the residents of New Orleans or other communities similarly afflicted with waterborne carcinogens, the low-level exposures become a day in and day out, day in and day out unrelenting series of cellular insults. For some people — we can never know in advance who they are — the accumulated carcinogenic burden becomes too great to handle. They become victims of cancer.

What is the measurable human toll? In the Environmental Defense Fund study, researchers compared New Orleans, which draws its drinking water supplies from the Mississippi River, with nearby Louisiana parishes, which utilize local ground water free of these carcinogens. They found substantially higher mortality rates from cancer of the bladder, kidney, stomach, and colon — the digestive and excretory organs — among New Orleans residents. Among white males alone, and only in New Orleans, researchers calculated that more than fifty premature cancer deaths each year were the consequence of drinking carcinogen-contaminated water.

Government testing undertaken in the aftermath of the Environmental Defense Fund study revealed that the problem was not local to New Orleans. Of the seventy-nine drinking water systems subsequently studied by the federal government, *all* of them — Philadelphia's, Cincinnati's, Miami's, Seattle's, and many more — contained significant quantities of cancer-causing contaminants. Liquid carcinogenic pathways. If the New Orleans experience is an indicator of the consequences of ingesting water laden with carcinogens, then the aggregate national cancer toll that is reasonably attributable to contaminated drinking water supplies may number many thousands of Americans each year.

Carcinogenic pathways. Atmospheric pathways. Human pathways. Liquid pathways. There is yet one more: the commercial pathway. Industrial production in the United States is not an exercise invented for its own sake. Its purpose is profit, and its method is to create and enlarge commercial markets. When the product is useful and has no serious adverse effects, the system can be a marvel of marketing efficiency. But when the product is discovered to have carcinogenic properties, the commercial pathways become insidious avenues of widespread cancer peril. Over the years, literally *billions* of aerosol spray cans were sold to the American people — hair sprays, hair conditioners, deodorants, indoor and outdoor pesticides — a major proportion of these jammed with vinyl chloride gas, a cheap, convenient propellant. The unwitting user inhaled up to 250 ppm of vinyl chloride gas in a single spray. Asbestos products, too, manufactured and sold by the thousands, have generally been marketed without serious thought to preventing the escape of the deadly fibers. Add to these the countless miscellany that is part of the modern American household: paints and varnishes containing trichloroethylene, a liver carcinogen; cleaning fluids and spot removers containing the leukemia-causing benzene or the liver cancer-inducing carbon tetrachloride. Gasolines, Adhesives. Polishes. The list is a long one.

The purpose here is not to instill fear of the carcinogenic pathways in our midst, but rather to emphasize that there are no reliable boundaries to check industrial cancer hazards. There are no sanctuaries. The relationship between industry and community is too intimate. The only rational protection rests in the development of sound social policies targeted to control cancer hazards at their source. This means a series of major steps. It means the firmest sort of no-nonsense policy to protect workers, because if the industrial workplaces of this land are engineered to be clean inside, it is less likely that cancer hazards will be carried outside. It means a massively increased enforcement effort by the EPA to immediately halt the dumping of carcinogens in the air and water. It means that the EPA must make maximum use of its authority under the 1974 Safe Drinking Water Act to adopt and enforce federal drinking water standards designed to purge the nation's water supplies of cancer-causing substances. And it means the most ambitious implementation of the Toxic Substances Control Act, systematically testing both old and new chemical agents in order to protect worker and citizen alike from the establishment of yet more pathways fraught with unnecessary cancer risks.

This kind of cancer control policy will entail major costs. But it would be a mistake to believe that a do-nothing policy is cost-free. On the contrary, the costs of doing nothing are enormous. Count the costs. Look first at the economic cost. Among its many ugly characteristics, cancer is a terribly expensive way to die. Typically, the disease involves costly treatments — surgery, radiation, chemotherapy — during a protracted period of worsening disability. There are often lengthy hospitalizations. A hospital stay generally averages sixteen days, and multiple admissions are very common. The direct costs for a particular cancer patient — for doctors and hospital care and therapies — may range from $5000 to over $20,000. Added to these costs are the indirect costs: the loss of earnings due to the illness itself and a foreshortened lifespan. According to the Third National Cancer Survey (1969–1971), these costs push the total dollar loss in a typical case of cancer to approximately $50,000.

Nationally, the aggregate economic cost of cancer exceeds $20 billion per year. But in addition to the sheer size of this loss, there is the question of its unjust distribution. Industrial plants responsible for occupationally and environmentally induced cancers rarely incur the costs of the horror they have created. The firm that dumps carcinogens in the Mississippi River at St. Louis never pays for the cancer-causing effects in New Orleans.

Even among workers struck with job-caused cancers, there is rarely compensation for their illness or death. The workmen's compensation laws are riddled with archaic provisions that make it difficult and often legally impossible to succeed with an occupational cancer claim. Like victims of environmental cancer, few workers can "prove" that carcinogenic exposures, which occurred years earlier, caused the malignancy. This is particularly true when the cancer in question is a common one like lung cancer, capable of being caused by a number of chemical agents. In this respect at least, Pete Gettelfinger was "lucky." His liver angiosarcoma was a cancer so rare and so clearly the product of vinyl chloride exposures that the legitimacy of his workmen's compensation claim was undeniable.

In Joe Fitman's case, though, his recovery of workmen's compensation benefits wasn't for job-caused cancer; the problems in proving the link between his lung cancer and what he breathed and worked with each day were too difficult to overcome. Instead, his attorney seized upon the "fortuitous" fact that Joe Fitman was also being strangled by emphysema, and it was on the basis of his less controversial claim of emphysema — not his cancer — that the companies involved agreed to settle.

The fact that Gettelfinger and Fitman were awarded any workmen's compensation benefits at all is exceptional. Usually, companies successfully avoid paying these financial costs. However, a cost is a cost. It is an expense incurred and someone must pay it. And, so, in this instance, the costs are incurred by the workers themselves — and their grief-stricken families. The medical bills pile up. A life's savings are exhausted. And then come the debts. What is taking place here, then, is a classic subsidy — a subsidy to industry paid for by the uncompensated victims of industry-caused cancer.

Tough, effective, preventive policies would have a twofold impact on national cancer costs. First, the overall costs would be eased as the incidence of cancer declined. And, second, those costs would be shared on a far more equitable basis. Vinyl chloride offers a useful example. When the federal government belatedly established its exposure standard of one part per million, a standard that will no doubt save many lives in the decades ahead, the government simultaneously forced the costs of cancer prevention — better equipment, better monitoring, tighter controls — back onto the major polyvinyl chloride producers. In this way, the expense associated with this strict cancer prevention standard becomes an added cost of doing business. Some of this cost is absorbed by the polyvinyl chloride producers, and the balance is passed along to wholesale and retail purchasers.

These, then, are the elements of cancer prevention: a reduced hazard; a reduced cancer toll; and the sharing of the immediate costs involved. *Sharing the costs in preventing cancer* — this is the key, and it is really the only ethical option in the face of the cancer pox. It is the only ethical option because the other costs associated with cancer — the biologic costs and the emotional costs — cannot be shared. Biologically, cancer is an all-or-nothing proposition. People are either struck by the disease or they are not. The luckless victims pay the ultimate biologic price while the nonvictims pay nothing.

So it is, too, with the emotional costs of cancer. Cancer. The Crab. As Alexander Solzhenitsyn wrote in *Cancer Ward,* " 'The Crab loves people. Once he's grabbed you with his pincers, he won't let go till you croak.' " Understandably, this is how many victims react to the disease. Cancer is a special kind of killer. To the victim, the malignancy is an invader of privacy. It violates the body's integrity. It destroys human dignity. It is a permanent trespasser haunting the victim with the specter of lingering death. Death by inches. This cost of cancer — the frightful toll it exacts upon the human mind and spirit — cannot be broadly shared. The victims, and those closest to the victims, pay all.

Part IV

Chapter 7.

Ruth Beaver

RUTH BEAVER IS SIXTY-FOUR YEARS OLD, her appearance unflattering. She is perhaps thirty pounds overweight. Her hair is short and styleless. She dresses in oversized muu muus. But still, her face is pleasant, her eyes large. She is warm and talkative. And it is easy to imagine that Ruth Beaver was once an attractive young woman.

Since separating from her second husband some fifteen years ago, she has lived alone. Hers is a simple existence. She gets by on a monthly disability check from the State of California, nearly half of it spent on rent for her small apartment in a deteriorating section of Hollywood. She passes her days tending to her limited needs — shopping, marketing, maintaining her apartment. And, now, riding on city buses to meet her medical appointments. Recently, Ruth Beaver had the lower lobe of her left lung removed. It contained two tumors — malignancies that were almost certainly the product of a lifelong smoking habit. Dating back to her years as a young girl in the mid-1920's, cigarettes have always played an important part in Ruth's life. They still do.

I was thirteen years old when I inhaled my first cigarette. The circumstance was — this little girlfriend of mine — I was thirteen and she was fifteen, and she had been smoking and she said, "Try it Ruth." Well, I did and I was so sick for three days. Yes, I inhaled and got sick and that was the end of it. That one puff. Maybe a couple of weeks later I tried the second cigarette. I still got sick. I took two or three puffs that time. But the third cigarette — that didn't bother me. We'd smoke — I'd go down to her house when her mother was gone — we'd smoke then. Or we'd go out — sheds they had in those days — and we'd smoke back there. Maybe I had two cigarettes or three or four a week. So that's how it started.

Teen-agers, you know, we were teen-agers. They all smoked. I'd buy the cigarettes myself. I looked older than my age, really. If I can remember I think they were Camels. In those days, you'd get two packs for a quarter. Then you could buy what they called a tin — fifty in a tin for thirty-five cents. I liked smoking. All the young people would smoke, all the younger crowd. All young people smoked cigarettes like they're smokin' pot now, I guess.

But it must have been offensive to the adults. It was looked down on, I guess, because I tried to keep it from my folks. Sometimes we'd smoke at my house. If my mom and dad would come home and smell cigarette smoke, my mom would say, "I smell cigarette smoke around here." And I'd say, "Well, I guess — somebody must have . . ." You know, I lied my way out of it, easily. And, you know, I'd chew gum and everything.

I was my daddy's favorite of the three girls — we were three girls. He just thought his youngest daughter — that was me — was so ladylike. And he was kind of old-fashioned. Well, one day when I was seventeen he came home unexpectedly. I had friends in — a girl that I went to school with — she and her husband were over visiting. And I was puffin' on this cigarette and when he came in, oh, golly, I thought, oh. It broke his heart. He said, "Put that cigarette out immediately and don't let me ever catch you with another one in your mouth!" Well, that was like saying — he should have known — that was like sayin', "Coffee table, move yourself." You know, it was like talking to a stone wall because I already had the habit since I was thirteen. I was addicted.

In those days no one spoke of addiction, or habituation, or cigarette-related health hazards. In the late 1920's and early 1930's, the mass production and mass marketing of cigarettes were still fairly new to the American scene. But it quickly became apparent that cigarette smoking was more than just another commercial phenomenon. Cigarettes held a special attraction for the young. Like automobiles, cigarettes were becoming a cultural craze. Puffing. Inhaling. Brand names. The arrival of cigarette advertising.

I smoked Luckies, Camels, Chesterfields. We'd change off, you know. We wanted to try 'em all! I think Chesterfields was my favorite in those days. They seemed a little milder.

1931 Blow some my way . . . It's a cool and comfortable smoke of milder and better taste. Chesterfield. They satisfy — that's why!

At one time I switched to Luckies.

1932 Do you inhale? What's there to be afraid of? Seven out of ten inhale knowingly — the other three do so unknowingly . . . And since you do inhale — make sure — make absolutely sure — your cigarette smoke is pure — is clean — that certain impurities have been removed! Lucky Strike. It's toasted.

Camels were awfully strong. But I smoked 'em when I got 'em free.

1934 Camels are from finer, *more expensive tobaccos* than any other popular brand. Camels. Smoke as many as you want . . . they never get on your nerves.

For some years after she was a grown woman — even after she was married to her first husband — Ruth lived at home with her parents in Indianapolis, Indiana. Despite her acknowledged dependence on her mother, she always held her own in terms of employment. Throughout the Depression she worked for the Indianapolis Parks and Recreation Department, organizing recreation programs for youngsters.

I lived home 'til mama died. I always lived at home. And my first husband — when we married — I said yes, but only if we can live at home. So, you see, I was a mama's girl. It was Depression time besides, now remember — 1932 — and so we all lived at home. Of course, by that time my mother knew I smoked and, oh, she still hated it. But my sister — the middle sister — she smoked and I smoked. My eldest sister, no.

In 1934, Ruth's father died of tuberculosis. It would be only the first of a series of family deaths caused by lung disease.

Yes, my dad died in 1934 of tuberculosis. He contracted that from the First World War. And when he came out they called it bronchitis. And later it developed . . . And he was in all the sanatoriums — government sanatoriums all over the place — through his veteran's benefits. My mid-

dle sister — now she was always kind of sickly and evidently she picked up the germ, I think, from him when he came home on a visit. She picked it up where I just had a stronger constitution. My middle sister and I were very close. Just inseparable practically. And she was dying. She died of TB at the age of thirty-three. The doctor gave her six months, and she died in six months and one week. She died at home. Sadness. I was heartbroken. Yes. Yes. And I would sit up with her. And so would my mother.

My sister had her little bell. And she'd ring and I'd take her bedpan. And I'd take care of her. My other sister was afraid of the germ, but I wasn't. We could see her go down. Weaker day by day by day by day by day. And she said to me — she called me Bitty — she said, "Bitty, don't let 'em put me in the sanatorium . . . Promise me. Promise me." I said to her, "No sanatorium. No sanatorium." And the doctor said it wouldn't do her any good if you put her in a sanatorium. They didn't have the drugs then they have now. She had cavities in both lungs the size of your hand.

She'd ring the bell. It wasn't always the bedpan. Sometimes it was 'cause she wanted company. And I'd sit there 'til I could see her getting drowsy. And she'd say, "Honey, you shouldn't be in here — the germ." And I'd say, "Baloney. Give me a puff off your cigarette." I'd make her feel like . . . Do you know what I'm trying to convey to you? Put her at ease. Make her feel like it was all right. She smoked right up 'til the day she died.

Day by day by day by day. Down, down, down, down. We were there right to the end. My sister said, "I want communion." So I called the priest and he came out and gave her communion. Three hours later she was dead. She closed her eyes and that was it. Of course, in our religion that was a wonderful thing. That was a great consolation to all of us. Yes, I was there. A tearful time, yes it was. I couldn't go to work for about ten days after her death. I wouldn't eat. Couldn't sleep. Seven months later my mother died of a heart attack — just a broken heart really.

With her father, mother, and middle sister dead, and her first marriage ending in divorce, Ruth was on her own. For her, World War II was a time of purpose and independence, a time of great personal pride. She was a part of a whole country going to war.

•

During the war, I would go around to different dance studios and we'd get our talent and we'd put together a show. We'd get paid for that. We'd go to Camp Atterbury in Indiana. We'd take shows out to the boys in training, and I'd emcee the shows. I thought I was, oh, so glamorous and oh, so — you know. And I guess I probably did a lousy job. But I was just conceited enough to think that I was good. And they, well, we always had a big crowd 'cause I had young girls. Real young, pretty dancers, you know. That drew 'em in. This was during the war.

The special officer – he got my cigarettes for me. Tareytons. I smoked almost exclusively those Tareytons during the war. They were hard to get, Tareytons. You couldn't even buy Tareytons. The boys were allowed the Tareytons. Herbert Tareytons they were called then. You know, the man with the little black hat. And so the special officer would get me my cigarettes, so I had nothing to worry about. No problems. All I wanted. Everybody smoked. Every woman I knew smoked. Really. E-v-e-r-y-b-o-d-y smoked.

After the war, Ruth married a second time and moved to Florida. Her husband was a steamfitter, and they lived in the Miami area. The marriage lasted eleven years before they separated and she moved to California. There, like her father and her sister, she found that she was afflicted with tuberculosis. During the 1950's, while recovering from the disease, she was confined to a TB sanatorium on several occasions. Interestingly, she smoked through it all, often with the approval of her physicians. Her life, her lungs, and her illness were increasingly entangled in the cigarette habit.

In the 50's I switched to L & M's. It was because of my chest condition. And I figured that the filter would get the tar. It's not the nicotine really that's bad on your lungs. It's the tars. There are enough tars in one cigarette to kill ten people really. It's true. So I figured, well, I'll smoke the filters. So I switched to L & M.

1958 Puff by puff today's L & M gives you less tars and more taste. L & M's patented filtering process electrostatically places extra filtering fibers crosswise to the stream of smoke — enabling today's L & M to give you — puff by puff — less tars in the smoke than ever before.

*I stuck with L & M's. But then I switched to a menthol brand. Alpines.
'Cause I got a coupon on the back every time I bought 'em. I was smokin'
Kools, which is a menthol. Then I saw the Alpines with the coupon and I
said, "Well, I'm gonna save 'em up." In fact, I've got practically a book
of 'em now. But then I quit the menthol. Someone said they're hard on
your stomach. I smoke Kent now.*

1959 It makes good sense to smoke Kent — and good smoking, too!

By 1974, Ruth had smoked a pack a day for more than fifty
years. More than 350,000 cigarettes. And, finally, lung cancer.

*I started feeling bad. I said, "There's got to be something wrong.
There's just gotta be something wrong. I can't get out of a chair. I can't
hardly pick up a cup of coffee." And I can't tell you how many chest men
I called. And none of 'em would take Medi-Cal* [California's medical
assistance program]. *None of 'em. None of 'em. None of 'em. "No, we
don't take Medi-Cal." "No, we don't take Medi-Cal." "No, we don't take
Medi-Cal." And I exhausted myself day in and day out. And then I called
Dr. Schneider* and asked her secretary if Dr. Schneider takes Medi-Cal.
And she said, "A few." And so she made an appointment, and Dr.
Schneider said for your first appointment you have to round up all your
x-rays. And I said, "Well, how am I going to do that?" And she said, "I
don't know. That's up to you. But you do it."*
*When I went in with my x-rays, we didn't even exchange greetings.
She just held up the x-rays. She said, "Will you go to the hospital for a
biopsy?" I said, "Sure. I'll go to the hospital for a biopsy." Well, I went
up there to Cedars of Lebanon and went through all their tests. And I
was there ten days before the surgery. They found two tumors in my left
lung — lower left lobe. But they weren't too large. Later they told me they
weren't sure if I'd make it through surgery. But I made it. I've got the
constitution of a horse. I think I was on the table six-and-a-half hours. It
was nip and tuck all the way. Nip and tuck. They didn't tell me that 'til
much later. But they could have told me. You're born and you die. You're
born and you die. I knew I had cancer when I went into the hospital. I*

---

*Dr. Rea Schneider is a Los Angeles physician specializing in pulmonary
medicine.

*wasn't scared. I had the priest come, and he gave me communion before
the operation. No, I wasn't afraid. I'm not afraid of dying because, you
know, there's a wonderment about it. What — you know — what we're in
for. No, death doesn't bother me. Now, maybe if Dr. Schneider told me
that tomorrow you're going to die, tomorrow at noon you're going to —
that will be it — you'll be dead, well, then, I don't know what I'd do.
Maybe — I don't know. But right now, no. I'm not afraid.*

*In the hospital, I had no desire whatsoever for a cigarette. I didn't
have my first cigarette 'til I came back home again. But then, when I was
home, I wanted one right away. But I didn't reach for it 'cause my niece
and her husband brought me home from the hospital. I could hardly wait
for 'em to get out — so I could have a cigarette! And when they said they
were going, I didn't say, "Well, why don't you stay longer?" Of course,
my niece could read me like a book 'cause she told her mother, my sister
Eleanor, "Aunt Ruth could hardly wait 'til Jerry and I were out of the
house so she could smoke a cigarette." While I was gone to the hospital my
sister and her husband came up and got all the cigarettes, you know. And
my niece found a package in the bathroom. I had a package in the bedroom, too, by my bedside. And before she left, my niece said, "Where else,
Aunt Ruth, that mother missed?" I said, "Honey, that's it." But I had 'em
anyway. But I didn't tell her that.*

*I'm not concerned about the cancer coming back. If it does, it does. I'm
sixty-four. I've led a pretty good life. I mean I haven't committed murder.
I've only hurt myself. I haven't hurt anybody else. I've never stole anything. I'm not a liar. I don't prevaricate. I procrastinate but I don't prevaricate. I've led a pretty good life.*

Ruth is a kind, likeable woman. Despite her troubles, she is
not a complainer. In fact, she is so genuinely humble that when
she finds people like her beloved Dr. Schneider, she gushes with
gratitude and is seemingly at a loss to understand how anyone
could be so dedicated to making her well again.

*I want to quit these cigarettes. I have to. It's Dr. Schneider — 'cause
she will not take me if I smoke. She said, "I'll kiss you off quick." That's
exactly what she told me. She said, "If you keep smokin', I don't want to
take care of you because I'm wasting my time." She's a dedicated doctor.*

*She went to a lot of trouble for me, and if I was to deliberately let someone
down like that — that isn't kosher. Oh, she's very serious! She's allowed
me six cigarettes a day because she knows that it's $275 to go to Schick*
[smoking cessation clinic] *— so Dr. Schneider knows that I can't go to
Schick right now. Lord help us, that Dr. Schneider! She is a doctor from
the top of her head to the tip of her toes. She means business and no
monkey business. And that's it — six cigarettes a day — that's all she
allowed me. She allowed me that 'cause between the diet for my weight
and the cigarettes, I was about to blow my head. But — she's not gonna
hear this — sometimes I smoke eight.*

*Yes, I'd quit these cigarettes tomorrow if I could. Of course I would! Of
course. You ask any heroin addict if he wouldn't like to quit and he'd say
yes. I think these are far worse. Oh, yes, I'd quit tomorrow. In fact, as
soon as I can, I'm gonna go to Schick because I want to quit. Of course.*

*I regret ever having taken that first puff. Oh, I most certainly do.
Ab-so-lute-ly! That first cigarette. But, you see, I'm gullible. I most certainly wish that I had never heard of a cigarette, never seen one. If I
could go back — I regret it, of course I do. And don't you ever dare
smoke. Don't you dare. 'Cause it can get to be such an agonizing thing. I
don't know how people quit cold turkey. Now, my friends, they quit.*

*I've got a weight problem, too. I told Dr. Schneider, "I'm goin' on a
Jewish binge — bagels and lox and cream cheese." She said, "Don't you
dare!" I love that lox and that bagel and that cream cheese. And God,
yes, that homemade cream cheese. There's a little delicatessen over near
here, and I slip over there and get those pickles and that other stuff. And
then I tell Dr. Schneider, "Well, I'm on a Jewish binge." And she says,
"Now, Ruth, I mean it. That's it. No more." And so I haven't. I'm losing
some weight and that's what satisfies her. She knows that I'm trying. She
knows. It's her. She's making me do it. Making me try to lose weight and
stop smoking. 'Cause I know if I don't I'll lose her. And I don't want to
lose her. She just means that much to me as a doctor, 'cause she's all doctor. And she is a wonderful doctor. And she is a dedicated doctor. And I
probably would have died without her. She spotted that tumor that quickly*
[snapping her fingers]. *We didn't even exchange greetings or names.
Nothing.*

*Now, would you look at that! This morning I counted out six cigarettes
and put 'em in that tray. And here it is only two o'clock in the afternoon
and I'm smokin' my sixth cigarette.*

•

Several months later, in early 1975, Ruth was hospitalized again. The lung cancer had metastasized, and there was a new tumor, this one lodged in her brain.

There was terrible pain and suffering. Only the application of the most drastic radiation and drug therapies brought any relief. After more than a month in the hospital, Ruth was home now. She had much to tell. But her voice had a very different, more anxious tone to it. It was almost shrill. Her account was both rushed and rambling, and riddled with ambivalence: expressions of fear and then displays of stoicism; expressions of hope for more time, and then a recognition that the end was near.

That's when it started — in February. I told Dr. Schneider — I said, "Dr. Schneider, there's something pullin' me down." So she made an appointment. And I kept gettin' down and down. I gave all my jewelry to my niece. I gave my sister anything that, you know, well, I thought I'll get rid of this apartment and I'll give the furniture to my great nephews. I just had no incentive. I just didn't care. Then something said, "Just hang on."

I called the doctor Sunday and I went into Cedars the following Tuesday. I was getting progressively worse. I didn't even pack. I just wore what I had on — a gown and a robe. I couldn't hardly walk. Right away, they sent me in for a skull x-ray and a brain scan.

I never went through such torture and hell in my life. I thought they were strokes. We all thought I was having light strokes. My mind was going like this: chug, chug, chug. My mind. I was blowin' my mind. I really was. I think I was ready for a nervous breakdown. I'd cry and cry all night long. I'd talk to myself. The nurses would come in and say, "Mrs. Beaver, were you talkin' to yourself?" I'd say, "No. I'm damn mad. I'm gonna put that damn light on." I was embarrassed, you know. And I couldn't help but talk to myself. And I do it right now, in this apartment. It must be from the medicine. I hope to God it is!

Dr. Schneider, she said, "You have a lesion, Ruth." She said, "A tumor. Cancer." Your brain swells and, oh, those headaches. I'd sit up in that lounge. In two weeks, I had maybe but one hour of sleep. I was fightin' that Demerol. I was fightin' that narcotic. I thought, "That's the last stage. If I have got to take morphine, I want to be able to take it for a while." Those headaches. There is nothing you can do for 'em. There's nothing. There's nothing. Nothing. You want to take and cut your head off. Like I told Dr. Schneider, I said, "If they told me they would cut my arm off without any anesthesia and my headaches would go away, I'd tell 'em to do it." That's how I felt. They're the most excrutiating headaches. There's nothin' can touch it. A migraine is just the tip end of it. This was from the brain tumor.

It wasn't until four days before I came home from the hospital that my headaches stopped. Nuclear medicine — that's what they put me on. And Decadron, which is a derivative of cortisone. The radiation is shrinking the tumor. And it's powerful. Oh, it's powerful. And I responded just like that [snapping her fingers]. *I tell you, it's my attitude that did it. I know. When you stew and worry about your condition — when you stew and worry and say, "Oh, I'm so sick." Well, I was sick, really. I didn't know how sick I was. Truthfully, I was a lot sicker than I thought. But knowin' it's cancer — that didn't bother me. Susan Hayward, you know, that's what she had — a brain tumor. They couldn't do surgery. You know, certain parts of the brain you can't do surgery. She was also at Cedars. God love her little heart, she suffered. Oh, at the hospital they said how she suffered. I said, "I know it. I know. I know. I have it." You become nauseated. And then these headaches. Oh! That's over with. Oh, and there's nothing you can do for it. Oh, my God, if there was just somethin' you could do for that nauseated feeling and the headaches with it. But none of it's . . . It's all gone. Gone. Gone.*

But really, I think I should have stayed in the hospital. But I was on the brink of a nervous breakdown, really. I really was. When you sit and cry like that and talk to people . . . I even made up people I talked to. Hallucinating. I'd draw my curtain every night. That was my little state room. Now I was ambulatory. One night I evidently had gotten warm and had taken my gown off and it had fallen by the bed. And I thought, "Now where in the hell am I?" And I went out in the hall stark naked — not a damn stitch on! The nurses all down the hall were laughin'. Miss Morris, my nurse, said, "Oh, Mrs. Beaver, I'll get you a gown." I said, "I don't care if you get me a gown or not." I said, "I don't need a gown!" I was oblivious of everything.

But when they started me on nuclear radiation, oh, I tell you, I just responded beautifully. Beautifully. I was upset a lot. The medication upset me. And Dr. Schneider had empathy for me. She knew. She knew what I was going through, you see. She is the most wonderful doctor. I love her. I absolutely, positively adore that woman. I really and truly do.

Now, I have a problem — this hair. I cried buckets of tears. Buckets and buckets and buckets when my hair started comin' out. Oh, how I cried and how I cried. So this little girl, Julie, came in to the hospital — in the bed next to me. She was thirty-one years old with cancer of the cervix, the back, the spine, the stomach, the throat. Thirty-one. And she has six children and five-year-old twins. Beautiful children. She said to her doctor, "You got me through '74. How much of '75 do I have?" He said "Julie, let's take it 'til July. I promise you 'til July. Then we'll take it from there." She said, "I've got to make preparations for my kids." Her attitude on life! And I said, "My God, I'm cryin' over six hairs on my head and this child is cryin' for time to make preparations for her family." I said, "Julie," I said, "if I could give you one second, honey, one minute of life, I'd walk from here to L.A. and go through Bullock's without a hat or a hair on my head." My attitude changed completely then. I said to Dr. Schneider, "I want to go home. I want to go to my little quiet apartment. It's not much, but I want to go home."

So I'm home now, and I've got Demerol here. And she has to give me a prescription for Percodan — pain pills. And phenobarbital — 100's. And I'm gonna keep only three of each and hide 'em — give the rest to my niece to give to her husband to lock up in a safe, 'cause if they knew I had that they'd break in here and cut my throat. My God, this neighborhood is horrible. It's horrible. I'm in bed every night at eight-thirty, listening to my radio — the talk shows. And I lock up real good. I had a dead bolt put on. And I leave my porch light lit all night. To hell with that electric bill. I'll do without something else. 'Cause they can climb in right off that roof — the roof off the patio.

Tomorrow's my last day on the radiation. So, now I'm going to find out if I can take Schick. Now, when I asked Dr. Schneider, she says, "Oh, I allowed you those six cigarettes. Take your six or eight cigarettes, Ruth. Don't spend your money on Schick." So, now I don't know what she's getting at by saying that, 'cause she's death on cigarettes. The cigarettes are hard on the heart and the blood vessels, and at my age it's one of the worst things I can do. They're nasty; they're dirty; they're expensive. But by smokin' I am not being fair to those doctors that have worked so dili-

gently to save my life. And then to do something that's tearin' me down. Right now I need the cigarettes. I need 'em. I really do. But when this is over, I'm going to do everything in my power, to the utmost, to quit. I'm not being fair to those doctors. How can a doctor help you if you're tearin' down what he's trying to build up? I'm addicted to cigarettes. Fifty years! I am so full of nicotine that I think even going to Schick won't do it. But I'm willing to try anything.

And when I get a little more strength and can get out on my own . . . I want to do some volunteer work. And, it's been ten years since I have put on make-up other than lipstick. I have never wanted to dress. I have muu muus. This was my attire for the day. A closet full of clothes, but I didn't care. Just let it go. Now I have incentive. I want one of my rings back. I told my sister, I said, "Honey, I'm an Indian-giver, but I will wear my ring now." They're just imitation diamonds, but they're very pretty. And she said, "Well, honey, I've had it put away for you, Ruth, hopin' some-day you'd take an interest. You always had so much pride. You were losin' your pride, honey. And you were always so pretty and I was so proud of you. And I'm so glad you're beginning to dress." Now I wear heels, you know. Haven't done that for ten years. My outlook has changed com-pletely.

Now, I had to buy a special bed so I can sleep with my head up. See, I can't lie flat 'cause I get a fuzzy feelin' — enough to keep me awake. Of course, I'm awake a lot. I'm tryin' to get off of sleeping pills. I'm not tak-ing any. And I didn't go to sleep until five this morning. I get about three hours every night. But I'm going to break that damn sleeping pill habit. I don't want to take those damn pills! I don't want to put that stuff in my stomach. There was a time when I needed it. I fought it in the hospital.

But, you know, I'm goin' out, not comin' in. Like I said, if I was a young woman, I'd probably be worried sick. But I'm not a young woman anymore. My fun is all behind me. I had a glorious, absolutely beautiful life. Dancing. Fun. Traveling all around. I had gaiety. I had a full, full life. I have no regrets. I'll be sixty-five in October. How many more years have I got? Maybe ten at the most. And in my condition, who knows? Well, I could live to be a hundred!

Oh, yes, I've got it licked. Oh, yes. Definitely. Oh, they wouldn't have released me from radiation if they didn't . . . Now have you noticed I held that cigarette? I didn't smoke it. Heavens, I'm gonna make it. If I do, I do. *If I don't, I don't. It's not worrying me. I'm not upset about it. Not in the least. I just want some energy so I can start goin'. I don't mean pell-mell. Now, I can get on this No. 89 bus that'll take me all the way down Hollywood Boulevard to Farmer's Market — for a dime. So you can't go wrong, can you? A dime for senior citizens. Senior citizens! Oh, God, I hate that damn word. I do look it, but I don't act it. I mean my thoughts aren't senior citizen. I think young, you know. Unless I look in that mirror, I'm still twenty-five. I'm still a beauty bird, you know. Oh, yes. I hope it doesn't change. Give me some life.*

Chapter 8.

Cancer for Sale

RUTH BEAVER died on September 16, 1975. From the time of the original diagnosis of lung cancer, the odds against her surviving were always severe. More than 90 percent of lung cancer victims are dead within five years. Few survive the disease because lung cancer ordinarily has no reliable early warning signs. The persistent cough, the bloody sputum, the chronic fatigue — these symptoms do not precede the development of a lung tumor; they generally follow it. And by the time the tumor is first seen on an x-ray, it has already reached sizeable proportions. Too much time has been lost: time for the malignancy to metastasize. Even before lung surgery is performed, cancerous cells are likely to have been carried through the lymphatic channels to new sites in the respiratory system; or, as in Ruth Beaver's case, the malignant cells may have gained access to the blood system and traveled to the brain and other organs, where they establish secondary tumors beyond the effective reach of conventional therapies.

The lung itself, where the biologic damage began, bears evidence of the savage abuse that led to the malignancy. Instead of normal, pink tissue, the interior of the smoker's lung is coated with a black, sticky residue. This is the "tar" in cigarette smoke — the particulate matter that remains after the tobacco has burned. Tar consists of hundreds of separate chemicals, some of them highly reactive agents that assault and injure successive generations of lung cells. Fortunately, the human body is not without its defenses in the face of this chemical onslaught. Recent research in immunology has noted the body's natural capacity to not only resist the cancerization process, but, some researchers say, to actually track down and kill cancer cells even as they develop. Remarkable though it is, the body's immunodefense system must be viewed realistically. Obviously, it is not fail-safe. Like an anti-ballistic missile system that theoretically might be able to explode ten or twenty or fifty offensive missiles, as the number of incoming enemy missiles increases to 100 or 200 or 500, the system at some point becomes overloaded and inadequate to meet the attack. So it is with the tissue in a heavy smoker's lungs. And so it was with Ruth Beaver. And so it was with more than 80,000 other Americans who died of lung cancer in 1975. Nearly all of them were long-time cigarette smokers. Most of them died at about sixty years of age. If they had not smoked, at least 80 percent of these people never would have been afflicted with lung cancer.

The traditional way of looking at cigarette-caused lung cancers is to see these premature deaths as essentially self-inflicted tragedies. Ruth Beaver's death, so the argument goes, was her own doing; her own choice; her own fault. At first glance, this explanation is as attractive as it is simple. The smoker's conduct is considered an act of self-destruction. The victim is blamed for the tragedy. And, by implication at least, all other parties are exonerated.

Popular as it may be, this view is dangerously misleading. It looks upon cigarette-caused deaths as somehow inevitable. It ignores the fact that human behavior, including an individual's decision to smoke or not to smoke, is influenced largely by deliberate governmental and corporate policies. This is not conjecture. It is historical fact. And the history is worth knowing if future governmental and corporate policies are to be directed toward cancer prevention instead of cancer promotion.

Lung cancer is now so rampant, its death net so wide, that few people realize that it was an almost unheard of disease before World War I. Dr. Alton Ochsner, who later played an important part in the cigarette controversy, recalls his own introduction to lung cancer dating back to 1919. At that time, while Ochsner was a junior in medical school at Washington University in St. Louis, a patient with cancer of the lung was admitted to Barnes Hospital, the teaching hospital for the University. In a short time, the patient died. Dr. Ochsner remembers the incident.

Dr. George Dock, who was an eminent clinician and pathologist, asked the two senior classes to witness the autopsy because, as he succinctly said, the condition was so rare he thought we might never see another case as long as we lived. Being very young at the time and enamored by the clinical knowledge and judgment of our eminent professor of medicine, I was greatly impressed by this extremely rare condition.

What Ochsner had in fact seen — "this extremely rare condition" — was the beginning of what would become, in his own lifetime, a national epidemic of almost unbelievable proportions.

After graduating from medical school, Dr. Ochsner went on to become a leader in lung cancer surgery. But in addition to his contributions as a surgeon, he was among the earliest scientists to explore the relationship between cancer of the lung and the use of tobacco.

Seventeen years elapsed before I saw another case of lung cancer, at the Charity Hospital in New Orleans after having come to Tulane University as Professor of Surgery in 1927. There was nothing particularly unusual about seeing a rare case in 17 years, but eight other additional cases were seen in a period of six months which was extremely unusual. Having been impressed with the extreme rarity of the condition 17 years previously, the sudden increase in incidence represented an epidemic, and there had to be some reason for it. All the patients involved were men; they all smoked cigarettes heavily and had begun smoking in the First World War. I then ascertained that very few cigarettes were consumed before the First World War but during the war and afterward there had been a tremendous increase. Since there was a parallel in the rise in sale of cigarettes and the appearance of the new disease with a lag of approximately 20 years from 1914 to 1936, I considered that this might be the necessary length of time for a possible carcinogenic agent in tobacco smoke to become evident. The evidence was admittedly very nebulous, but it seemed as if this was the most likely cause.

Just as Ochsner and other scientists began to consider the connection between cigarettes and cancer, another group of professionals — advertising executives — embarked upon their own mission: harnessing the new commercial technology — radio as well as print media, to cultivate a potentially enormous national market for cigarettes. The selling began.

> 1929 An Ancient Prejudice Has Been Removed. Gone is that ancient prejudice against cigarettes . . . The "TOASTING" has destroyed that ancient prejudice against cigarette smoking by men and women. Lucky Strike. "It's toasted."

But Luckies offered more. There was a better life ahead through cigarettes, and a very special message for women; the lurking shadow, the shadow of overweight that stalks every woman, could be avoided. Refrain from overeating.

> 1930 When Tempted, Reach for a LUCKY instead.

Health fears? On the contrary. The commercials made it sound as if cigarette smoking were actually a requirement for good health.

> 1936 Smoking Camels stimulates the natural flow of digestive fluids . . . for Digestion's sake . . . smoke Camels.

In 1913, when Ruth Beaver was three years old, cigarette advertisers spent $13.8 million peddling their wares. By 1925, when she was fifteen and hiding her smoking habit from her parents, the annual advertising had jumped beyond $20 million. Throughout the Depression of the 1930's, cigarette advertising increased, reaching an estimated $50 million in 1940. Annual per capita cigarette consumption — the total number of cigarettes sold in a year divided by the number of Americans fifteen years or older — rose steadily. In 1913, per capita consumption amounted to 163 cigarettes for each American adult. By 1925, per capita consumption reached 690 cigarettes. And fifteen years later, in 1940, the figure was 1828 cigarettes. Typical of the latent period associated with carcinogens, the widespread use of cigarettes that began with World War I later reflected itself in an accelerating cancer toll. Records show virtually no lung cancer deaths among Americans in 1913; 2357 deaths in 1930; and 7121 in 1940.

Prior to the outbreak of World War II, a number of European studies indicated a strong statistical association between lung cancer and smoking. Then, in 1941, Alton Ochsner joined with Michael DeBakey, the now-famous heart surgeon, in publishing the first American study to stress the cigarette-lung cancer connection. Based on clinical observations of autopsies performed in the United States and in other countries, these researchers found that the incidence of pulmonary carcinoma — malignant tumors situated in the surface tissue of the lung — had doubled over a period of eighteen years. Meanwhile, the increase of all other malignant tumors noted in the autopsies had been slight. Citing the parallel increase in cigarette sales over the same period, their study concluded, "It is our definite conviction that the increase of pulmonary carcinoma is due largely to the increase in smoking, particularly cigarette smoking, which is universally associated with inhalation."

The Ochsner-DeBakey study received scant popular attention. Like other scientific reports bearing upon public health, its findings were generally under-reported. Probably less than one in 10,000 Americans ever heard of the Ochsner-DeBakey study. But in contrast, during that same period, just about every citizen within earshot of a radio knew that "Lucky Strike Greens [had] gone to war!" A cigarette going to war? It seems that early war shortages made it difficult for the American Tobacco Company to secure the dyes necessary for the traditional green and gold Lucky Strike package. What loomed as a marketing setback was turned to quick commercial advantage when Lucky Strike adopted a dyeless white package — and its memorable patriotic slogan. And, so, during the early months of World War II, when each Saturday evening millions of Americans sat by their radios tuned to the Hit Parade, they heard the mellow voice of Andre Baruch gravely announce, "Lucky Strike Green" — (pause for a trumpet blast and a drum roll) — "has gone to war!" Later, with the color transition safely made, Lucky's promotional message changed again. By 1945, probably half of the American populace knew what "L.S.M.F.T." meant: "Lucky Strike Means Fine Tobacco."

Despite the clever slogans and the multimillion dollar saturation campaigns, the smoking-health issue was attracting increasing interest in the scientific community. Shortly after World War II, the cigarette controversy emerged as the major concern in cancer epidemiology. Interestingly, amid an atmosphere conducive to scientific inquiry, Washington University in St. Louis contributed more than its fair share of prominent personalities to the cigarette-lung cancer investigation. Of course, Dr. Ochsner was himself a graduate of Washington University. But there were others. Dr. Evarts Graham, who in 1933 performed the first successful pneumonectomy for cancer of the lung, was Alton Ochsner's professor of surgery in his senior year. Some years after his graduation, when Ochsner first argued that the increase in lung cancer was due to cigarette smoking because of the parallel between the sale of cigarettes and the increasing incidence of the disease, he was chided by Graham. Graham, himself a very heavy cigarette smoker, said, "Yes, there is a parallel between the sale of cigarettes and the incidence of cancer of the lung, but there is also a parallel between the sale of nylon stockings and the incidence of cancer of the lung." Ochsner remembers more.

A few years later Dr. Graham wrote to me and reminded me [of the incident] and said that he would have to "eat crow" because a young man, a sophomore student at Washington University, had taken his (Dr. Graham's) cases of cancer of the lung and studied them and the results of the study convinced Dr. Graham that there was a relationship between cigarette smoking and cancer of the lung. This young sophomore student was Ernst Wynder . . .

In 1950, Wynder and Graham together published the results of their large-scale epidemiologic study. In their investigation, they employed a retrospective method: they interviewed patients already known to have lung cancer and, inquiring about their smoking habits, they then compared these responses to the responses of patients without lung cancer. The results indicated that proportionately more heavy smokers were found among the lung cancer patients than the control group population. Wynder and Graham concluded: "Extensive and prolonged use of tobacco, especially cigarettes, seems to be an important factor in the inducement of bronchiogenic carcinoma."

Persuaded by the evidence, Graham altered his smoking habits, decreasing his cigarette consumption to six per day — two after each meal. In 1953, when Wynder and Graham were able to prove that the tar from cigarette smoke produced skin cancer when applied to the surface of animals, Graham quit smoking altogether. But it was too late. He wrote to Alton Ochsner, "Because of our long friendship, you will be interested in knowing that they found that I have cancer in both my lungs. As you know, I stopped smoking several years ago but after having smoked as much as I did for so many years, too much damage had been done." Two weeks later, Dr. Evarts Graham, the first person to surgically remove a cancerous human lung, was himself dead from lung cancer.

In 1953, 23,502 Americans lost their lives to lung cancer. In that same year, per capita consumption was 3562 cigarettes, sustained by cigarette advertising expenditures that had soared to levels over $100 million per year. With the escalating human toll and the mounting scientific evidence, the cigarette-lung cancer connection at last began to attract some degree of publicity in the national press. In 1952, the *Reader's Digest* printed an article entitled "Cancer by the Carton." While the article represented an important breakthrough and registered a sizeable short-run impact upon cigarette consumption, it evoked a response from the industry that would become a familiar pattern during the course of the cigarette controversy: with each new disclosure linking cigarettes to cancer, the industry stepped up its advertising campaigns, trying to drown out the adverse message and at the same time encourage more smoking. Responding to what they branded a "health scare," cigarette advertisers concocted a new propaganda barrage that promised both smoking pleasure *and* good health. And now it could all be *seen* on television — persuasive visual images of carefree, safe smoking. Seventy-eight million dollars went into television advertising in 1957.

More doctors smoke Camels than any other cigarette.

L & M — Pure White Miracle Top of Alpha-Cellulose (just what the doctor ordered).

Meanwhile, in scientific circles, any major doubts about the cigarette-cancer connection were largely laid to rest by a series of impressive studies concluded in the mid-1950's. The most influential study was undertaken by Drs. Cuyler Hammond and Daniel Horn. With the assistance of American Cancer Society volunteers, Hammond and Horn conducted a so-called prospective study. They tracked 187,783 men, who were apparently healthy, to determine what effect, if any, smoking habits would have upon their mortality rates in the years ahead. The results, published in 1958, confirmed the findings of smaller, previous studies: among those who had died, a disproportionate number were cigarette smokers. In fact, cigarette smokers were dying at a rate approximately 70 percent higher than nonsmokers. Lung cancers and cancers of other sites accounted for a disproportionately high number of the excess deaths. In the Hammond-Horn study, as in all the major studies undertaken in the 1950's, another common finding surfaced: as the amount of cigarette consumption increased, so did mortality rates. An especially significant finding — with important implications for public health policy — was that the mortality risk from smoking decreased as the number of years of smoking cessation increased.

By 1960, a scientific consensus on the causal connection between cigarette smoking and cancer was clearly evident. The cigarette, first described as possibly "associated" with lung cancer and, later, as a "factor" in the disease, was now described with increasing confidence as the overriding cause of the twentieth-century lung cancer epidemic. Surveying the cancer carnage in 1961, Dr. J. Clemmensen, a highly respected Scandinavian epidemiologist, was moved to remark: "It seems impossible to escape the conclusion that we are now facing one of the major catastrophes in medical history."

"One of the major catastrophes in medical history." In 1961, 38,929 Americans died of lung cancer; per capita consumption hit 4266 cigarettes; and cigarette advertising surpassed the $200 million per year level. Two years later, in 1963, the statistical read-out was grimmer yet: 43,568 dead of lung cancer; per capita consumption at 4345 cigarettes; and cigarette advertising expenditures of over $249 million. The media drive had turned into a commercial cacophony. Visual and lyrical images abounded: virile young men and seductive young women romping in the outdoors, their bliss seemingly made possible by the ubiquitous cigarette. Is there any wonder that each year two million American teen-agers were becoming habituated to cigarettes?

What's it like to smoke an Alpine? Well, it's like many fresh little things you enjoy. It's like the breeze through the willows at the waters [sic] edge — or the way the air feels at dawn . . . a bright, invigorating taste . . .

Clean and fresh as all outdoors — that's the pleasure you get in the clean fresh taste of Belair.

Come to where the flavor is . . . Marlboro Country.

In 1962, as the tripartite juggernaut — advertising, consumption, and lung cancer — continued to gain momentum, Dr. Luther Terry, Surgeon General of the United States, appointed a prestigious committee to examine the evidence on smoking and health and to report its findings to the American people. In January 1964, the Surgeon General's ten-member Advisory Committee on Smoking and Health released its definitive study on the cigarette controversy. After an analysis of the scientific evidence pertaining to the lung cancer question — animal studies, clinical studies, and epidemiologic studies — the committee reached its most important conclusion:

Cigarette smoking is causally related to lung cancer in men; the magnitude of the effect of cigarette smoking far outweighs all other factors . . .

But there was more to report. The committee's work triggered a flood tide of incriminating data.

• Average cigarette smokers are nine to ten times more likely to get lung cancer than nonsmokers.

• There is a dose-response relationship between cigarette smoking and lung cancer. As with exposure to other cancer-causing agents, those who have smoked for many years, those who have smoked heavily, and those who have regularly inhaled deeply are at sharply greater risk than the lighter smokers. Heavy smokers are at least twenty times more likely to get lung cancer than nonsmokers. One in five heavy smokers dies of lung cancer.

• Because women tended to take up the cigarette habit later than men — the great surge in women smokers came during and after World War II — the 1960's would mark the beginning of a second huge wave in the lung cancer epidemic, with women representing an increasing proportion of the overall lung cancer toll. Lung cancer claimed the lives of 5163 women in 1960; 10,536 in 1968; and 17,262 in 1974.

• While occupational exposures to carcinogens and the carcinogens present in urban air pollution are also causative factors in lung cancer, in terms of numbers of deaths, cigarette smoking is nevertheless the preeminent cause of the lung cancer epidemic. In fact, the evidence indicates that cigarettes can interact with occupational and urban carcinogenic influences to actually *multiply* the lung cancer risks. Asbestos workers who smoke cigarettes experience this synergistic effect. While asbestos workers generally incur lung cancer at a rate seven times that of the general population, those asbestos workers who smoke are *ninety-two* times more likely to die of lung cancer than men who neither work with asbestos nor smoke cigarettes.

• Specific carcinogens present in tobacco smoke include benzo(a)pyrene, dibenzo(a,i)pyrene, and several other polycyclic hydrocarbons, as well as arsenic, DDT, cadmium, and other known cancer-causing agents.

• Smoking causes not only lung cancer but other cancers and other diseases as well. Smokers are more likely than nonsmokers to die of cancer of the lip and mouth, cancer of the larynx, cancer of the esophagus, bladder cancer, kidney cancer, stomach cancer, and cancer of the pancreas. They are also far more prone to die prematurely of heart disease.

With the release of the Advisory Committee's report on January 11, 1964, the purely scientific phase of the cigarette controversy had largely run its course. Almost immediately, the controversy shifted to the political realm: a clash between public health considerations on the one hand and private economic interests on the other. The stakes were evident from the outset. The mere issuance of the Surgeon General's report, coupled with the attendant publicity, produced a short-run, one month decline in cigarette sales of nearly 20 percent. The industry's response was predictable. In addition to denying the validity of the Surgeon General's findings, manufacturers pumped still greater expenditures into television advertising. In the spring of 1964, Morgan J. Cramer, Jr., President of P. Lorillard and Company, proudly reported at the company's annual shareholders' meeting that "April sales of P. Lorillard and Company are running ahead of last year's following a 'low point' in February — thanks in part to record levels of advertising." Cramer continued, observing that the decision to respond to the Surgeon General's report with increased advertising "had already been proved sound — by the turnaround in sales."

Cramer's corporate colleagues apparently agreed, because in the one-year period following the release of the Surgeon General's report, they increased television advertising alone from a level of $151 million per year to over $170 million per year. And in the four-year period from 1964–1967, cigarette advertising on television soared by 50 percent. The strategy produced a commercial cascade of jingles and jangles so pervasive that to this day — more than a decade later — the words in the advertising messages seem to leap off the page in catchy little tunes forever imprinted in the minds of tens of millions of Americans.

Winston tastes good like a cigarette should.

You get a lot to like with a Marlboro. Filter. Flavor. Pack or box.

You can take Salem out of the country but — you can't take the country out of Salem.

In spite of its lasting damage to the public's health, the industry's lyrical overkill did not alter the fact that the Surgeon General's report, unlike less influential reports that preceded it, could not be buried by silence. Its most valuable contribution was that it made cigarette policy a matter of national debate. Prior to 1964, Congress did nothing of consequence in the cigarette field except to quietly foster the growing of tobacco and the sale of tobacco products with hefty agricultural and marketing subsidies: nearly $20 million in 1955, rising to about $40 million in 1963.

In the winter and spring of 1964, after the release of the Surgeon General's report, Congress was not required to act in response to the findings. In fact, it is likely that no congressional action at all would have been forthcoming had it not been for the maverick conduct of the Federal Trade Commission. Citing the Surgeon General's report, and then citing its own statutory responsibility to regulate commerce in order to eliminate unfair and deceptive trade practices, the FTC proposed a regulation that required in every cigarette advertisement — radio, television, billboards, and print media — and on every pack, box, and carton of cigarettes, the prominent inclusion of one of the following warnings:

(1) CAUTION — CIGARETTE SMOKING IS A HEALTH HAZARD: The Surgeon General's Advisory Committee on Smoking and Health has found that "cigarette smoking contributes substantially to mortality from certain specific diseases and to the overall death rate";

or

(2) CAUTION: Cigarette smoking is dangerous to health. It may cause death from cancer and other diseases.

The fact that the regulation required a warning statement on every pack, box, and carton of cigarettes was not nearly as significant as the requirement that the warning accompany any advertising, including broadcast advertising. A disclosure statement of the kind proposed by the FTC threatened to destroy the appeal of radio and television advertising.

Remember some of the television ads of the day: for example, the Winston commercial showing a man and a young boy sitting in a disk-sled, spinning and twisting down a snow-covered slope. When the man tumbles off the sled, a woman — presumably his wife — happily brushes the snow off his clothing, and they both reach for a Winston. Then, the pitch:

> Find folks who know the knack of having fun . . . and chances are, you'll find Winston. It figures, because this cigarette delivers flavor twenty times a pack. There's a pure snow white filter here of course, but it's what's up front that counts — and up front is Winston's exclusive Filter-Blend. Filter-Blend means choice, golden tobaccos specially selected . . . and specially processed for filter smoking. And that means smoking at its flavor-filled best! Discover for yourself why, when all is said and done, this one quiet fact stands out . . . more people smoke Winston than any other filter cigarette, because Winston tastes good like a cigarette should.

Now, imagine the devastating impact of hearing next the short, sixteen-word warning proposed by the FTC:

> CAUTION: Cigarette smoking is dangerous to health. It may cause death from cancer and other diseases.

No amount of visual "fun" could overcome the shock effect of the words "death" and "cancer."

In 1964, the industry was pumping nearly four-fifths of its $261 million advertising budget into radio and television. Faced with the pending FTC regulation, the tobacco lobby — those who grow, manufacture, or sell tobacco products — turned to Congress for help. Congress dutifully responded by passing the Federal Cigarette Labeling and Advertising Act of 1965. In this act, Congress blocked the FTC's proposed regulation and required instead that as of January 1, 1966, all cigarette packages, boxes, and cartons sold in the United States must bear the statement: "Caution: Cigarette Smoking May be Hazardous to Your

Health." Beyond this inconspicuous side-panel requirement, the Congress refused to compel the industry to include the mildly worded warning in radio and television advertising. Radio and television, at that time the very key to the promotion of cigarettes, were left untouched. In fact, the labeling act expressly prohibited the FTC and state or local agencies from taking any action to require health warnings in advertising for a period of four years. The entire apparatus of federal, state, and local regulatory authority was suspended in exchange for the nine-word side-panel warning.

Though the warning label was sure to be ineffective in discouraging smoking, it had an important legal implication. Lawyers for the major cigarette companies actually advised their corporate clients of the benefits of the label. Increasingly, cigarette manufacturers were facing lawsuits filed on behalf of longtime smokers who had died from lung cancer. Each lawsuit claimed that cigarettes were responsible for the lung cancer death and that the victim had never been warned of the product's dangers. Fearing a rash of successful suits, the lawyers for the cigarette manufacturers advised that with the new legislation they could point to the label as adequate warning, at least sufficiently adequate for the purpose of cutting off any future legal claims.

As expected, when the labeling requirements took effect on January 1, 1966, there was no significant impact on cigarette sales; per capita consumption increased in 1966. The selling and killing went on as before. The entire episode characterized the first time — but not the last — that Congress intervened to block an emerging anticigarette policy that promised success, only to substitute its own predictably unproductive approach.

Shortly after this major setback at the hands of Congress, health educator Dr. Milton Terris wrote of the failure to bring about a reduction in cigarette smoking:

> The reason for failure is that individual health behavior, like all other behavior, does not occur in a vacuum; it is conditioned by past history, by the entire economic, social, and political structure of society. The feeble attempts at health education on cigarette smoking [such as the

side-panel label] are reminiscent of Don Quixote tilting at windmills; how much effect can they have in competition with the estimated 300 million dollars of miseducation per year paid for by the tobacco companies?

Discouraged though he was, Terris's thesis — that health education can work, that patterns of individual conduct can be changed for the better as well as for the worse — was about to be proved correct. In mid-1967, one year and a half after the labeling act became law, a startling development occurred. A young attorney, John Banzhaf III, filed a petition with the Federal Communications Commission, the agency responsible for licensing radio and television broadcasters. In his petition, he called upon the FCC to make a finding that cigarette commercials were really statements depicting just one side of the smoking controversy and, that under the FCC's "Fairness Doctrine," stations were required to provide equal time for the presentation of the other side of this important health controversy. In a landmark decision, the FCC agreed with much of Banzhaf's argument and obligated stations to accord a "substantial" amount of air time — although not equal time — to the "other side" of the cigarette controversy.

This ruling launched the nation on a three and a half year experiment in public health education by way of anticigarette commercials. Affirmed by the courts in 1968, the FCC action was interpreted to mean that radio and television stations had to provide roughly one anticigarette message for every five procigarette messages. Translated into aggregate terms, this meant that by 1969 and 1970, approximately $40 million per year in broadcast time, free of charge, was given to the American Cancer Society, the Tuberculosis Association, and other nonprofit organizations to present hard-hitting anticigarette messages. It was a unique era in broadcast advertising, giving rise to a host of creative anticigarette advertisements. For example, there were the short "I Quit" messages with Tony Curtis, Tony Randall, and others. Or the parody of the Marlboro man: a tough-looking, gun-toting cowboy pushed his way into a saloon, inhaling a cigarette; he began coughing uncontrollably and was pushed aside by a clean-cut, nonsmoking cowboy. Then the word "cancer" zoomed up on the television screen followed by the announcement, "Cigarettes — they're killers."

Perhaps the most forceful of the anticigarette messages on television was the one in which William Talman, the actor who played prosecutor Hamilton Burger on the Perry Mason series, introduced his family and revealed that he had lung cancer. He urged smokers to quit and nonsmokers to never start. By the time this particular anticigarette message was televised, William Talman was dead from lung cancer.

During the years 1967–1970, the Banzhaf decision had a major impact on cigarette consumption. After years of virtually uninterrupted growth in per capita consumption, there was a slight fall-off in 1967: 4280 cigarettes for every American eighteen years of age and older, as compared with 4287 in 1966. In 1968, per capita consumption fell again: to 4186 units. In 1969, when FCC monitoring and public pressure were assuring widespread compliance with the Banzhaf decision, anticigarette messages were in full swing; and per capita consumption suffered its most severe drop-off, down to 3993 units. In 1970, a further decline was registered, down to 3985 cigarettes. The American people were participating in a demonstration of the effectiveness of mass media public health education (see the graph on p. 134).

From 1967 through 1970, an unprecedented 10 million Americans, mostly adults, quit smoking.

Although the FCC facilitated the era of anticigarette messages, this novel venture in public health education had its beginnings in the private, not the public sector. Indeed, both in its origins and in its content, the anticigarette campaign was almost exclusively a product of the private sector: a private attorney filed the original Fairness Doctrine petition; most of the required antismoking messages were actually produced by various private health agencies — the American Cancer Society, the American Heart Association, and the Tuberculosis (now Lung) Association; the broadcast time itself was a $40 million per year involuntary donation by radio and television stations across the land. Contrasted with this private activity, the federal government's investment in the production and distribution of anticigarette messages never exceeded $1 million per year. If ever there was a backdoor entrance to a successful anticigarette policy, this was it. Quite by accident, it seems, the nation had stumbled upon a creative, noncoercive, anticigarette campaign that was working. And working well.

The anticigarette messages proved two things: first, that broadcasting alone is an effective instrument of public health education, even with a physically habituating substance like cigarettes; and, second, that a sustained campaign in the broadcast media has sustained impact in depressing cigarette consumption.

Left alone, the anticigarette media campaign seemed destined for a long and successful life. Each year, cigarette advertisers could be expected to buy hundreds of million of dollars in broadcast time; and, under the force of the Fairness Doctrine, anticigarette messages would continue to be aired because of the prevailing five-to-one formula. But, then, in 1969 Congress reentered the picture. The four-year termination date on its 1965 legislation was drawing near and, seizing this opportunity, Congress intervened in the cigarette controversy for the second time, enacting the Public Health Cigarette Smoking Act, which included two principal provisions. First, in a minor concession to the mounting scientific evidence concerning the destructive effects of cigarette smoking, Congress changed the cigarette side-panel label from "Caution: Cigarette Smoking May be Hazardous to Your Health" to "Warning: The Surgeon General Has Determined That Cigarette Smoking Is Hazardous to Your Health." The second principal provision in the Public Health Cigarette Smoking Act was a ban on radio and television cigarette advertising effective January 2, 1971.* Although the cigarette manufacturers felt obliged to oppose the radio-television ad ban as product discrimination, their opposition was strictly a

---

*Congress chose January 2 instead of January 1 to allow one final blast of advertising on New Year's Day when Americans by the tens of millions were watching the football bowl games. Cigarette companies spent $2.2 million in television advertising on that last day.

token gesture. Privately, they actually favored the pending legislation, because they believed that a radio-television advertising ban would serve to undo the anticigarette campaign that was only possible because of procigarette advertising. With the banning of procigarette commercials, stations would no longer be legally bound to present the "other side" of the controversy.

Some health-oriented congressmen expressed concern over this point and sought assurances from the radio and television broadcasters that they would maintain the millions of dollars worth of anticigarette advertising. While spokesmen for the stations pledged that they would continue to air a heavy volume of anticigarette messages, Congress never wrote such a requirement into the law. It was a foolish error.

If there is a cardinal rule in regulating the American corporate economy, it is this: where the pursuit of private profit conflicts with the public good, it is naive to rely upon the promises of corporate voluntarism. The only reliable means of ensuring the keeping of such promises is through the force of law.

On January 2, 1971, cigarette advertising was finally off the air. But, beginning that same day, anticigarette messages virtually vanished from the scene. The country's three and a half year experiment in mass-media antismoking education was finished. Meanwhile, in 1971, cigarette promoters managed to shift $150 million of their more than $200 million per year in radio-television expenditures into other outlets, principally newspapers, magazines, and billboards. The effect of all this upon per capita consumption was as dramatic as it was predictable. After a historic four-year decline in cigarette consumption, an upward trend returned in 1971. In that year, per capita consumption rose to 4037 from the previous year's 3985. In 1972, the figure went to 4043; and in 1973 leaped sharply to 4147 (see graph on p. 134).

The FTC was so alarmed at the renewed upsurge in per capita cigarette consumption that it repeatedly advised Congress to allocate funds to the Department of Health, Education and Welfare to enter the marketplace and purchase radio and television time for anticigarette messages and effectively reestablish the health education program. The response from Congress: silence.

Annual Per Capita Cigarette Consumption*

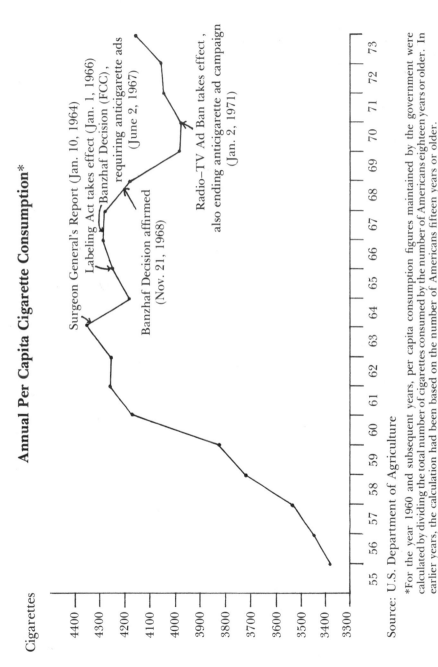

Source: U.S. Department of Agriculture

*For the year 1960 and subsequent years, per capita consumption figures maintained by the government were calculated by dividing the total number of cigarettes consumed by the number of Americans eighteen years or older. In earlier years, the calculation had been based on the number of Americans fifteen years or older.

In 1905, George Santayana, the renowned Harvard philosopher, observed, "Those who cannot remember the past are condemned to repeat it." But there is a more positive side to Santayana's proposition: namely, those who *can* remember the past may *choose* to repeat it. Certainly, in seeking to establish a national cigarette policy geared to public health instead of private profit, a wise course would be to choose to repeat history.

The 1967–1970 experience should have shattered once and for all the myth of programmatic helplessness in the face of the cigarette-cancer calamity. If the experiment accomplished nothing else, it proved that private decisions regarding cigarette smoking are susceptible to educational influence. This should come as no surprise. Cigarette advertisers would not have purchased $225 million per year in radio and television time unless they were convinced that their messages could influence behavior. And, quite naturally, these ads did influence behavior. Similarly, anticigarette messages worth $40 million per year in broadcast time also influenced behavior. It does not take a lawyer, or statistician, or social scientist to draw the appropriate conclusion: the Congress should immediately reestablish an antismoking media campaign comparable in scope and content to the 1967–1970 campaign. Since prosmoking messages have been banned on radio and television, free access through the Fairness Doctrine is no longer available. But, by legislation, Congress could either appropriate funds — about $100 million per year — for HEW to purchase radio and television time for anticigarette spots; or, it could mandate the networks to set aside broadcast time — perhaps a total of two minutes of prime time each evening — for anticigarette messages.

But congressional responsibility does not stop here. Government subsidies to those who grow and market cigarettes should be repealed in their entirety. While some subsidy programs have come under attack in recent years, the government still spends about $50 million annually on tobacco subsidies, roughly one-third of this amount used to market cigarettes abroad under the "Food for Peace" program.

On top of these subsidies is the biggest and best hidden subsidy of all: the tax deductibility of cigarette advertising. Consider the economics of the matter. A profitable cigarette company is likely to be in a 48 percent corporate tax bracket. This means that when it advertises its cigarettes and deducts the entire cost of the advertisement as an "ordinary and necessary business expense," the government — the American people — wind up paying for 48 percent of the advertisement. When, in 1970, cigarette advertisers spent $314 million, the American people paid for over $100 million of this cost in the form of lost tax revenues because of the deductibility of cigarette advertising. When, in 1970, Liggett & Myers launched a multimillion dollar campaign to promote its new women's cigarette, Eve, the public paid for nearly half the cost of the commercial claptrap invented by a few advertising executives.

> Farewell to the ugly cigarette. Smoke pretty. Eve. Hello to Eve. The first truly feminine cigarette. It's almost as pretty as you are. With pretty filter tip. Pretty pack. Rich, yet gentle flavor . . . Women have been feminine since Eve. Now cigarettes are feminine. Since Eve.

Congress is not required to grant tax deductions willy-nilly. Tax deductions are a matter of legislative grace and they should be authorized by statute only where there is at least a semblance of social benefit from promoting the product. There is no semblance of social benefit in the promotion of cigarette smoking. Quite the contrary. When a product is so demonstrably habituating and lethal, and when its social benefits are nonexistent, it is preposterous for Congress to provide a costly tax subsidy that actually spurs the peddling of these cancer-causing wares.

There is still more that the Congress must do. For many smokers, the cigarette habit is simply too strong, and quitting is too difficult. But steps can be taken to reduce the cancer hazards, even for these people. For instance, the government could discourage the production of higher tar cigarettes. Here, again, theory and actual studies show us that the carcinogens present in tobacco tar, like other carcinogens, exhibit a dose-response relationship. Reducing the dosage of the carcinogens will reduce, though not eliminate, the cancer risks. Even lifelong smokers like Ruth Beaver want to do *something* to lessen the risks:

> I figured that the filter would get the tar . . . It's the tars . . . It's true. So I figured, well, I'll smoke filters.

Public policy should encourage the switch to the production of less hazardous cigarettes by taxing them on a differential basis: higher-tar, higher-risk cigarettes should cost at least ten or twenty cents a pack more than the lower-tar, lower-risk brands. To further encourage the beneficial social trend of switching to less hazardous cigarettes, Congress might consider retaining the tax deductibility of cigarette advertising promoting brands with very low tar content.

An effective anticigarette policy will always be opposed by the tobacco lobby. Who could expect otherwise? It is indisputable that tobacco is, today, the basis of a multibillion dollar American industry. But despite the admitted size of the enterprise, tobacco production and its subsidization have always been a bad bargain for the American people. It costs the nation dearly in both economic and human losses. While there can be no compromise with the cancer pox, political wisdom suggests that there will be no positive gains in curbing cigarette consumption unless anticigarette measures include an interim policy to finance the transitional needs of selected segments of the tobacco industry. In addition to the large producers, there are in the United States several hundred thousand small tobacco farmers whose lives and livelihoods are tied to tobacco. Their interests should not be ignored. The answer is not to sustain and nurture a death-dealing industry, but rather to provide special transition subsidies to support farm income as tobacco farmers convert their efforts to growing soybeans and other crops more appropriate to a world beset by food shortages and a nation wracked with cancer.

If the past is to be an effective guide in fashioning a national anticigarette policy, it must be understood that strategy is as important as substance. The tone and tactics of a renewed drive for a national anticigarette policy must be carefully considered. Obviously, the purpose is not to design a punitive policy, prohibitionist in tone, and inclined to indulge in the fantasy that the smoker is a sinner who must be saved. Nor is the purpose to erect a policy of paternalism, complete with thousands of bureaucrats to hold the hands of American smokers. What is needed is not a holy crusade, but a disciplined, effective national program that can, and will, bring about a major reduction in cigarette-caused cancer deaths at a minimum national cost.

About 35 percent of adult Americans smoke. Almost 35 percent of America's teen-agers take up the habit, many of them destined to become the lung cancer victims of the first quarter of the twenty-first century. Without a strong national anticigarette policy, the country faces the continued squandering of human resources on a scale that no nation can afford. The bottom line, then, is really a fundamental issue of conservation. Conservation of human resources.

Federal health officials have estimated that a properly directed national effort should be able to produce a one-third reduction in cigarette smoking in just five years. The cancer deaths prevented by such an achievement would, in time, reach into the tens of thousands annually. The unnecessary loss of life to premature heart disease would also be sharply curtailed. As for those who might argue that government sponsorship of selected economic measures and a media-based, anticigarette campaign is somehow offensive, let's be clear about precisely who might take offense. Those most offended would be the powerful economic interests reaping huge profits from cigarette sales. The overwhelming majority of private citizens, however, can be expected to react favorably to this kind of anticancer public health program. In fact, surveys indicate that even among smokers themselves, half state that they *want* to quit smoking, just as Ruth Beaver wanted to quit.

In some ways, cigarette-caused cancers are among the most discouraging cancer cases, tied as they are to a contrived lifestyle pattern shared by tens of millions of Americans. Yet, there is a hopeful aspect to this, too. Because of its lifestyle origins, and because of the huge number of victims involved, cigarette-caused cancers provide the most promising area for public policy to cheaply accomplish a substantial reduction in future cancer deaths. Moreover, evidence suggests that cigarette consumption is not the sole area where cancer is tied to lifestyle. Several recent surveys of the cancer mortality among Mormons have found that, as a group, Mormons incur cancer at a rate of 25 to 35 percent less than in the United States generally. The preachings of the Church of the Latter-Day Saints strongly urge its members to abstain from the use of tobacco. But the lower cancer rates among Mormons cannot be explained by the avoidance of cigarettes alone. Apparently, another Mormon stricture — the stricture against alcohol — plays an important role, too. Cancer of the esophagus is caused not only by smoking, but even more so by heavy drinking. It seems that alcohol, which literally bathes the esophagus as it flows down a drinker's throat, acts as a carcinogen on esophageal tissue. Heavy drinkers succumb to cancer of the esophagus at a rate several times that of the general population. Among Mormons, however, esophageal cancer is a rarity, occurring 66 percent less frequently than in the general population. Similarly, primary liver cancer, another alcohol-related cancer, occurs among Mormons at a rate less than half that of the national average.

The experience of a second religious group, the Seventh-Day Adventists, provides important insight into what is, in part, yet another lifestyle cancer: colon cancer. Cancer of the large bowel. Each year colon and rectal cancer kill more than 50,000 Americans. Among women, these malignancies kill more than 25,000 each year, running a close second to breast cancer. But among Seventh-Day Adventists, the incidence of colon and rectal cancer is sharply less than in the rest of the population. The religious practices of Seventh-Day Adventists include a prohibition against eating meat, tending to corroborate the recent evidence indicating that the standard American diet, which is unnecessarily high in meat and animal fat, has a carcinogenic effect as it moves through the digestive system.

In still another diet-related area, it is now well established that women who are seriously overweight are prone to endometrial cancer — the most common cancer of the uterus — at a rate at least 50 percent greater than would ordinarily be expected. Apparently, obesity causes an increase in the production of the hormone, estrogen, that, in turn, poses a heightened cancer risk.

The estrogen-cancer connection developed a new twist when it was recently revealed that synthetic hormones, taken by tens of millions of menopausal and postmenopausal women, have led to a dramatic increase in uterine cancer. Spurred by overblown promises that estrogens could keep women "feminine forever," since the early 1960's a large percentage of gynecologists have been prescribing estrogen therapy for virtually all of their menopausal and postmenopausal patients — on an indefinite basis. Drug companies have cashed in on this commercial bonanza, with sales soaring to about $80 million annually. But that was before the 1975 studies indicating that women using Premarin and other synthetic estrogens are developing endometrial cancer at a rate as much as fourteen times greater than women who are nonusers.

Paralleling the Premarin boom of the 1960's was the advent of oral contraception. The pill. Promoted as both safe and effective, the pill became an implicit invitation to a new, freer sexuality. Millions of American women were placed on daily doses of contraceptive steroid hormones, their physicians giving scant consideration to possible long-term health effects. It is still too early for a definitive evaluation of the benefits and costs associated with this vast experiment in chemical contraception, but the emerging evidence is disturbing. In addition to the heightened risk of stroke and other dangerous disorders caused by blood clots, there are now clinical and epidemiologic data pointing to a possible cancer peril, too.

Writing in the *Journal of the American Medical Association,* three surgeons and a pathologist from the University of Louisville School of Medicine reported their observations of an increased frequency of primary liver tumors among women patients. They described thirteen patients — all of them pill-users — whom they saw in the period 1968–1974. They noted that in reviewing their tumor registry, no primary liver tumors had appeared in a comparable age group of women during the previous thirteen years. Of the thirteen patients reported, nine had so-called benign tumors; "benign" only in that they were not malignant, but nevertheless life-threatening because of the likelihood of hemorrhage. The other four patients with liver tumors had malignant growths. Three of these women died from the disease. Two were twenty-five years old; one was forty-seven. Citing findings similar to their own, the doctors noted that, in Iowa and elsewhere, clinicians were encountering what appeared to be an increased incidence of both malignant and nonmalignant liver tumors in young women. They concluded: "The etiologic role of contraceptive pills remains unproved, but a possible link between these pills and hepatic tumors seems increasingly likely."

This report followed a recent California study in which researchers described an apparent connection between the use of oral contraceptives and an increased risk of cancer of the breast. The added risk seemed to be among women who used oral contraceptives for two to four years, and among women with prior indications of benign breast disease. The investigators also reported an apparent increased risk of breast cancer in women who had taken the pill prior to their first pregnancy.

At this time, it is not possible to venture even a tentative judgment on the scope of the cancer threat posed by the pill. In the final analysis, perhaps looking back from the vantage point of the year 2000, it may be determined that the experiment worked out reasonably well. But meanwhile, the chilling fact remains that 10 million American women of childbearing age are currently taking the pill. In light of what is known, and considering all that remains unknown, this degree of national dependency on chemical contraception seems recklessly excessive.

Cigarettes. Alcohol. Diets excessively burdened with animal fat. Obesity. The indiscriminate use of synthetic hormones. The rush to chemical contraception. This should not be mistaken as a call for the establishment of a Spartan lifestyle as a matter of national policy. But to the extent that cancer is a product of commercially influenced lifestyle patterns — and in large measure it is — isn't there some responsibility to communicate this information to the American people?

Contrary to the cynical view held by too many in positions of high authority, the American people are neither dumb nor uninterested. They *do* care about their own health. They *do* care about the health of their parents and children. If they are properly informed, a sizeable percentage will try to maintain standards of good health. Their 1967–1970 response to anticigarette advertising proved the point. But who is to bear the message? If the government is not to be the messenger, then who is? Surely, it is not beyond the bounds of reason or constitutional propriety for the federal government to underwrite and sustain a noncoercive educational program emphasizing the causes of cancer and encouraging Americans to adopt a more moderate, less cancer-prone lifestyle for themselves and their families.

Part V

Chapter 9

Jennie Day

POLLY DAY is a nurse. Her husband, Julian, is in the insurance business. They were married in 1951 and, during the next fifteen years, they had five children. Their second daughter, Jennifer, was born on July 15, 1955. She died on November 4, 1967. The cause of death was a medulloblastoma, a fleshy gray tumor that compresses the brain stem, obstructing the flow of spinal fluid to the brain. The malignancy later spreads throughout the central nervous system.

Polly: Her name is Jennifer, but we used to call her Jennie.

Julian: She was different than our other children. She was a little different from most kids. I would say she was a little more tense than most kids. Very precise. She was an excellent student in school, an exceptional sort of person.

Polly: She really liked school. Did very well, from kindergarten on. And tried very hard. This is where the tenseness comes in. If she didn't do something as well as, say, her friend Cydney, it bothered her a lot. She was tense. She was a mature child for her age. And a very responsible girl. But she had a lot of fun. She was well rounded. She had a lot of friends at school and enjoyed and liked her friends.

Julian: She was a very physical child. She used to go like hell. She'd outrun everybody. A very wiry child.

Polly: She could even outrun her older sister.

When she was ten years old, Jennie's otherwise normal childhood began to go awry.

Julian: She started vomiting in the morning. We thought she had the flu. She'd get sick — every so often she'd get sick like she had the flu. I don't think she had any headaches or anything like that. It was like a stomach flu.

Polly: *Always in the morning. Since then I've learned that the pressure* [from the tumor] *builds up during the night, and then you vomit in the morning. And then she'd be fine, you know. You'd think there was nothing wrong with her. I'd keep her home and make sure she was okay, and then she'd go to school the next day. She never had a temperature. And when she did this — like twice — I took her to the doctor, and he checked her out, and everything was fine. And then the third time I called him again, and he goes, "Oh, gosh." He was frustrated. He didn't know what it was. And so he referred us to a pediatrician who started a more vigorous work-up.*

The medical people were beginning to suspect that something else was wrong. She was losing weight. And then we put her in the hospital, and they thought, well, maybe she had an obstruction in her intestines. Of course, once we put her in the hospital, and they started doing all of these various tests on her, then she really lost weight. She couldn't eat and then she'd vomit more and more — all the time – from increased cranial pressure.

She was in the hospital for six weeks before she actually had her surgery. At one point they were all set to do abdominal surgery on her. And they called the surgeon in and they did more x-rays, and he said there's nothing wrong there. And so then they called in a neurosurgeon and that kind of frightened us. He did a spinal tap and found an elevated protein in her spinal fluid, which indicates that something's going on upstairs that shouldn't be there. That's when he told us that they suspected that she might have a brain tumor, and that was really scary.

Next, they scheduled a pneumoencephalogram, where they inject air into the canal in your spine, and it's supposed to go up into your brain, and they x-ray that, and it outlines . . . But the first one didn't work out well. I think the tumor was blocking the flow of the fluid. So the air wouldn't go up. She got very sick during that thing. It was just an awful experience for her. Then they scheduled arteriograms where they inject dye into her neck — which they don't do anymore. They do it down in your groin now. But her neck was all . . . it was really painful.

Julian: *She put up with the tests. But it was miserable. You know, everything they did was painful. I don't know how she was able to take it. But I know it was rough on us too. I'd hate to see a kid go through all those tests again. I'll be frank with you, it's just so painful.*

Polly: She'd say to us: "What are they going to do to me next?" "Why don't they leave me alone?" "When am I going to get out of here?" It was awful. But she put up with it. I don't know how she did it. She was very adult for her age. These kids seem to almost develop a sense of adulthood.

Nothing was indicative of where the problem was, even though they knew there was something wrong somewhere. And in the meantime, of course, we were all in a state of anxiety. You know, we'd ask, "When is she coming home?" And, we could see she was getting worse. She looked like a little skeleton by this time. So then they decided they'd do one more pneumoencephalogram. We had a conference with the neurosurgeon and the pediatrician; the neurosurgeon said she's getting much worse, and we've got to do something. And he was going to drill burr holes in her head and inject the air that way. Well, it turns out that they tried it the other way first — through her spine — and they got through. They saw the tumor. And then they scheduled her for surgery three or four days later.

I just knew when they started looking for it . . . I just had a feeling, you know. It's intuitive. Something's bad; something's awful; it's there. They're not going to ever get it out. And I just knew that she wouldn't make it. And so she had her surgery. And the outlook from that was very bleak.

Julian: They didn't know it would be malignant until they actually saw it. At least, that's what they told us. And, of course, we were hoping that it wasn't. When he came out of the surgery, he told us — it was the worst.

Polly: He was very frank about it. I give him a lot of credit. He told us she tolerated the surgery well. And he told us what the tumor looked like, and, unfortunately, that it looked like a bad one. They grade them one through four, and it was a grade four. They're highly malignant. He told us that they would be giving her radiation treatments and that the life expectancy was probably about two years, although he had one child that lived four years. They took out what they could, but it evidently was attached to the medulla, so he couldn't really get it out. And he said that these things did seed into the spine. I think he was really very honest, for what we could absorb at that point.

Julian: The surgery left her with a partial paralysis. She kind of lost the function of one of her eyes. It kind of went off to one side, and she walked with kind of a limp.

Polly: Yes, she developed what they call a Bell's palsy from one of the cranial nerves. The surgeon felt that one of the cranial nerves must have been attached to the tumor so that when he cut it . . . when he went in there and took it out . . . He was upset with that. After that she had kind of a crooked smile, and one eye wouldn't close all the way. And then the gait problem; and she listed a little bit, too, afterwards.

When the surgery was over, she was not really told of the gravity of the situation. I think this is one of the regrets that I have. But at that time people just didn't do that. You know, now people are told, you know, "You have a cancer . . ." or whatever the kid can understand. And doctors try to make it more optimistic and are much more encouraging. At that time, we didn't have Dr. Ablin.* We got him later. He tried to talk to her, but she wouldn't really open up to him. And he wouldn't tell her either.

Julian: I still don't see the point in telling a child — at that point when they have another year or year and a half to go. I don't see where it does any good.

Polly: Well, they usually don't tell them right away. They tell them that "it's very serious and we're very worried about you, and you have this thing that might come back. But with all this treatment, you know . . ." And that's the way they usually go about it with children. But at that time we just thought, you know, we were going to be the big brave people and just make life go on naturally. Which, of course, it never did.

Right after her surgery she didn't have a sense that her condition was terminal. Not then, I don't think, because she continued to get better. She came home from the hospital around the Fourth of July, 1966, and her sister was born about two days after she got home. And she was really . . . Jule stayed home with the kids . . . and Jennie was cleaning around here and working and helping him.

We had a home teacher for her for a couple of weeks, and she absolutely hated it. So we got rid of the home teacher and she went back to school half day. And then later she went all day.

---

*Dr. Arthur Ablin is a pediatrician practicing in the San Francisco Bay area.

Julian: I know when she got well for a while, you kind of forgot about everything. You think, "Gee, she's getting better." And when she went back to school, you actually got to feeling like she's going to be all right. She almost looked like she was going to make it back.

Your hopes go up and your hopes go down. It's just continual, right from the beginning. You're up and you're down. You know, when they first found that it was a tumor, your hopes went down. Then they said it might not be a bad one, and your hopes go up. And then they come back and you get the worst — it's the worst. And you're down again. And, God, I can't tell you how many times we were up and down.

You're always hoping that they're going to come up with something new at the last minute. You always have that hope, which is kind of futile, I guess. But it's something to hang your hat on for a while.

Polly: The rest of that year was all right. We got through Christmas all right. And then it was April — almost a whole year — and then she developed increased cranial pressure from the scarring of the radiation and surgery. I kept her home from school and took her to the doctor, but I didn't realize then how bad she was. She really had bad intracranial pressure and she was talking nonsense syllables. So the doctor put her in the hospital right away, and that's when they did the shunt on her. They decided that she needed to have a shunt put in. The spinal fluid wasn't really moving. After she had the shunt done, they had to redo the shunt. Then they sent her home.

She was home one week, and, all of a sudden, she became paralyzed and she couldn't walk. She couldn't even hold her legs together. At first we thought she was just weak, you know. So then we took her in to the neurosurgeon's office, and he says, "The tumor has seeded into her spine" — at least that's what he thinks. And he sends her back into the hospital, and they do this myelogram [x-rays of the spinal cord after injecting a radiopaque substance]. *And they found out . . . sure enough . . . there it was. So he went in and did a laminectomy — he took off the top part of the vertebrae. He couldn't take the tumor out because it was attached to the spine, and if he pulled it off he would really foul her up — she wouldn't have any bladder function or bowel function. So he just did the best he could and left room for it to grow without causing any pressure. She came home again in July 1967. She was in the hospital about another six weeks. And while she was there, she kept asking: "What next?" "Why is everything happening to me?" And, of course, we knew we were on a downhill grade.*

And then they radiated her. When they got down to her back with the radiation, then she would get sick. She'd vomit.

Julian: Even the drugs she was taking — they'd make her face fat, you know, like a leukemia patient. It must have been particularly tough for her when she was going to school like this. And she had to wear a wig. It must have been difficult. I really used to wonder if it was worth it all — to put her through all of this.

I know during this period I worked all the time. Actually, I was better off working than sitting around here thinking about it. I had people say, "How can you work? How can you do things with this going on?" I just felt I was better off working than sitting around thinking about it. But, you know, it's never out of your mind. We just went along and did our work as best we could and tried not to think about it. But it was always there. I think it was harder on Polly than me because she was home with Jennie all day and I was away working.

Polly: It's there. I mean there's no doubt about it. But it didn't ever get to the point where we felt we were overtreating her until one doctor decided he was going to try some chemotherapy on her, and he started giving her vincristine. And I know he really wanted to do the best he could for her, but he really shouldn't have done it. That gave her problems. The side effects of vincristine were constipation, vomiting, and pain in the jaw and shoulder. The constipation was very bad. And then her blood count got so down. My God, she just didn't have any platelets left.

When we brought her home for the last time, of course she was already paralyzed. Jule bought her a hospital bed, and we fixed up her brother's room for her. And she stayed home from July until November, when she died. That was the best part, really, the idea that I promised her — I said, "No, you don't ever have to go back to the hospital." So she stayed at home. Just having her come home and die at home was considered a big pioneering deal.

Julian: She just hated the hospital so much that it was really a blessing to have her come home.

Polly: She was happy to be home. I think she felt so much better at home. Jule fixed up the TV in her bedroom. And we'd go in there and watch TV with her. Or her sisters and her brothers would be in there and they would bug each other — more like a normal . . .

She was paralyzed, but we'd get her up. We took her to the doctor's office. My dad would come over, or Jule would be here. And then Dr. Ablin would come to see her. Her paralysis was from the waist down — from the pressure on the spinal nerves. But she did have bladder and bowel function. She didn't have to have a catheter, which was good.

She did a lot of school work at home.

At night she'd have to be turned every two to four hours, so I'd have to get up and turn her. Then, in the morning, you know, we'd fix breakfast, and she'd either have breakfast in her room, watching the TV, or else we'd get her up in the wheelchair and she'd come in the kitchen. Then I'd give her a bath and change her bed and she'd be out in the wheelchair for a while. But then she'd get tired and want to go back to bed.

Maybe some little girl might come over to visit. She stayed in touch with her close friend, Cydney. And her other friends would send her letters and write her cards. A lot of people were always coming around and calling. Fortunately, we had a lot of good friends and a lot of support from neighbors.

After lunch, she might go back in her room and take a nap. Then in the evening Jule would come home and, since it was in the summer, we'd sit around outside and he used to mix us drinks, and she'd want peanuts — peanuts and drinks stuck out in her mind. And then we'd have dinner and try to, you know, figure out something that she'd want to eat. And the evenings were pretty much, you know, watching TV or whatever. Her spirits varied — some days up, some days down.

Julian: She got pretty disgusted with her state of affairs. She hated being confined to bed like that and seeing the other kids running around, doing all sorts of things.

Polly: She'd get depressed about that. She became very depressed when she no longer felt that she was going to get better and that her legs wouldn't return. Her weight was pretty good, but she never got back that muscle tissue that she lost. She used to have solid calves in her legs — from all that running. She never got that back.

Julian: Polly was giving Jennie the shots that she needed.

Polly: We both learned to give shots, although Jule didn't want to do it, *so I did it. And she was scared, you know, when we went in there and she needed something for pain and she said she didn't want me to give it to her. "No, no, no." she said. And after I gave her the first shot she says, "Gee, that wasn't so bad." And that kept her comfortable.*

But seeing your child wither away . . . it's awful. There's nothing quite like it. There isn't . . . I don't know of anything like it. Nobody knows how you feel except somebody who's in the same boat.

Julian: You just feel like throwing everything in the air and getting the hell away.

Polly: And then she wouldn't eat. You know, people who have cancer often just can't eat. They just feel so sick and lousy. They don't want to eat. So she became very dehydrated, and then she became more uncomfortable. So Dr. Ablin said, "This won't prolong her life, but we'll give her IV's just to get more fluid in her system." And it did; it made her rest better and a lot more comfortably. So he hung a hook into the wall for the IV bottle. He showed me how to do it. He'd start the IV's and we'd regulate them. He showed me the bottles and how much an hour he wanted to run. He came to the house with a whole box of IV bottles. He was really very supportive, I think.

At that point, I'm sure she knew she was dying. She just . . . she kind of withdrew. I know she'd say, "I'd just be better off not here." You know, things like that. You just knew she didn't even want to be here because she felt so rotten and she couldn't do anything that the other kids could do. And, of course, she'd complain of pain. She would say, "Why does everything have to happen to me?" And I found it very difficult. I'd like to talk to her about it without crying, you know. I didn't want to cry. I wanted to be really strong. Which probably isn't the greatest thing, either.

With something like this, I think you go through your grief from the moment you hear that your child has cancer. That's when your grief starts. So, by the time they die, it's . . . it's, you know. And I was going through a very religious period at the time. Well, I'm Catholic, and the kids have gone to parochial school. Of course, I became more religious when this happened. I mean, you know, "God's the only one that's gonna help me." I thought it was supportive. It was supportive for me. And Jule didn't quite go along with that. You know, "How could there be a God when all these horrible things are happening?"

Julian: I've never been religious myself. And I think I turned further away from it at that point. I felt if there is such a thing as a God, how could they do something like this to a little child.

Polly: I think it was kind of hard on my folks. My parents would come around and help a lot. It was hard on them. But it makes the grief afterwards much easier because we could plan. We had a real . . . a joyous funeral for her. It was kind of all planned in advance. Jule did all of that, too. Dr. Ablin suggested this — he came around and he said, "You had better start preparing because you shouldn't wait until the last minute." So Jule went around to all the places, and he picked one in San Rafael. And he made all the arrangements in advance. He even went down to the cemetery and picked out the plot. It was hard for us to discuss at that time, but yet we did it. We managed.

A nun brought me a record of folk masses. And I played it for Jennie and she picked out songs that she liked. We decided that we would have a folk mass. That was one of the first ones that was ever done. And it became a joyous type of thing — if you're a Christian, death is supposed to be the beginning and not the end.

She was kind of sleepy off and on before she died. She had been slowly going downhill for some time. Dr. Ablin had said — he came on Halloween and we made those pumpkins — and he said, "I really think she's going to die within the next few days." Then he came back the next day and said, "Gee, I'm really surprised. She's actually a little bit better than when I was here yesterday." You could arouse her, but she really wanted to sleep.

The day she died, Jule had gone someplace with the kids, and when he came back I said, "I really think she's kind of comatose." But you could arouse her. That was Saturday morning. My parents had been coming over every other day to help. And they were here that Saturday. They were going to have dinner with us. And I went in to turn her over before dinner . . . and she died. I called Jule from the other room, and he was there when she died.

We called the doctor and the doctor came. He was really good, too, with my parents. He came in the living room and sat and talked with them. It was very peaceful. It was really a peace. We were so tired.

Julian: It's funny. When you know it's inevitable that she's going to die, you just hope it will be soon. It was really a relief when it was all over. It was really a relief seeing her out of her pain.

Polly: Actually, I think when she died it was like somebody lifted a great weight off your shoulders. It was really peaceful.

But, of course, we think about Jennie often. And the children — we all think about her and talk about her and laugh about this and that. And, of course, we always go up to the cemetery all the time. I think about her all the time. Most of them are good, happy thoughts. I think the hard times are when you see . . . like her good friend Cydney. Cydney's grown up . . . she's a young woman . . . and she's going to college. That's the hard part. That's the hard part . . . when you think of what your child would be.

Chapter 10.

Childhood Cancers

CHILDREN WITH CANCER. It sounds strange, even awkward to those accustomed to thinking of cancer as an affliction that only strikes adults. Yet, in the United States, cancer is second only to accidents as the leading cause of death for children under fifteen years of age; and cancer kills more children between the ages of three and fourteen than any other disease. Each year, there are more than 6000 new cases of childhood cancer; annual deaths number about 3000. While leukemia remains the most common form of childhood malignancy, tumors of the brain and central nervous system — like Jennie Day's medulloblastoma — claim nearly 1000 lives per year. Other cancers, virtually unheard of among children, now appear to be cropping up in clinical reports with increasing frequency. A recent review of referral records at St. Jude Children's Hospital in Memphis, Tennessee, revealed a very worrisome increase in "adult-type" cancers in children. Of particular concern was the referral of nine youngsters with colon cancer in a brief fifteen-month period from 1974 to 1975. In the thirteen years prior to these referrals, there had been only four children referred with this type of cancer. Seven of the nine recent patients were from the same region and were reared in rural environments. Although unprepared to draw any final conclusions, the researchers at St. Jude point out that "the admission of nine patients with carcinoma of the bowel within a fifteen-month period is highly suggestive that there is an increasing frequency of large bowel cancer in pediatric patients and that environmental circumstances may have had a major role in the development of this tumor in these young patients."

Children with cancer. How does it happen? In many instances

— we cannot say for sure which individual cases — the cancerization process is essentially the same as among adults. Children are exposed to one or more environmental carcinogens in sufficient doses so that the accumulated biologic insults transform normal cells into cancerous cells. Depending upon the carcinogen involved, the result may be cancer of the bone, cancer of the kidney, or cancer of the brain. Perhaps the result will be leukemia: cancer of the marrow. Or lymphosarcoma: a type of lymphatic cancer.

The latent period that normally precedes the actual onset of a malignancy — ordinarily ten to thirty years — has its exceptions. For example, carcinogens that attack the blood-and-lymph-forming tissues, such as x-rays or various solvents containing benzene, can have a considerably shorter latent period. These potentially fast-acting carcinogens, when combined with the rapid cell division that is taking place as young bodies grow, seem to be capable of telescoping the cancerization process into the first five or ten years of a child's life. Julian Day recalled that, as an infant, Jennie had a heart murmur and underwent numerous diagnostic tests. At this point, years after her death from cancer, he can only ask the nagging questions; he cannot supply any certain answers.

When they diagnosed this heart thing with her, they ran her through a battery of tests and x-rays and all kinds of things. I've often wondered if all of that x-ray business could have had anything to do with the brain tumor. I've often wondered that because she had quite a number of x-rays. And fluoroscopy. I guess we'll never know if that had anything to do with it.

X-rays and fluoroscopy. These sources of radiation are well-recognized carcinogens that can cause various types of cancers, including both solid tumors and nonsolid malignancies, such as leukemia. Recent statistics indicate that, on an average basis, nearly half of the radiation exposure incurred by Americans is from medical or dental diagnostic sources. (Sunlight is the principal environmental source of radiation and is responsible for most skin cancers.) As with other carcinogens, the effects of radiation exposure are cumulative. The dosage from a single x-ray may appear relatively innocuous. But with each x-ray the risks pile one on top of the other, in some instances triggering a malignancy.

Although the hazard is now very well documented, too many medical and dental practitioners either discount or disregard the danger. In treating children, they too often forget that carcinogenic exposures constitute lifelong biologic burdens capable of developing into cancer at some unpredictable point in the future. They cavalierly order series after series of x-rays. Some do so slavishly, unthinking converts to the technology of radiography. Others do so out of sheer greed. Still others order x-rays in self-defense, as protection against potential malpractice suits. Whatever the reasons, unwarranted x-rays trade short-term convenience against long-term cancer peril. For the luckless youngsters who become the victims of radiation-caused cancer, the day of reckoning comes early in life.

As with cancer-causing agents in other contexts, the overriding objective of national policy should be to protect infants and children to the greatest degree possible by eliminating all unnecessary carcinogenic exposures and by reducing unavoidable exposures to an absolute minimum.

The record on needless radiation exposure is not encouraging. Nor is the record elsewhere. In March 1975, Dr. Irving Selikoff, who did the pioneering work on asbestos-induced cancer among insulation workers, provided a stark example of the laxity of federal policy as it relates to carcinogenic risks among children. According to Selikoff, his researchers had tested nineteen commercial baby and body powders. Nine of the products were found to contain asbestos fibers in quantitites ranging from 2 percent to 20 percent. In addition to asbestos-contaminated talc, many of the powders also included major quantities of nickel that, like asbestos, causes respiratory and other cancers. The question for future policy is a simple one: Are these sweet-smelling, carcinogen-laden products worth the cancer risks to tens of thousands of American infants?

Baby powders are an important source of infant exposure to asbestos-contaminated talc, but there are others too. Talc, like asbestos, is a mineral fiber and, like asbestos, its uses are myriad:

in roofing materials and in ceramics; as pigment in paints and varnishes; as filler in rubber, plastic, and paper; and also in products and processes intimately associated with childhood. Inflatable toy ballons are dusted on the inside with antistick talc powders. So are candy molds. And talc is commonly found in both "baby" aspirin and vitamin tablets.

An estimated 2 percent of rice sold in the continental United States — and almost all the rice in Puerto Rico — is coated with glucose and talc, a process permitted by the FDA, although coating is likely to result in talc and asbestos residues on the rice, even after washing it. Coating adds no nutritional value to rice and apparently has but one purpose: to make the uncooked grains look glossier and more attractive, hence more saleable. In large cities like New York and San Francisco, coated rice is sold mostly to people of Spanish or Oriental extraction, who, of course, take it home and eat it. And feed it to their children.

A similar display of FDA footdragging involves the food additives sodium nitrate and sodium nitrite. Nitrate and nitrite are used to preserve ham, bacon, frankfurters, luncheon meats, and smoked fish. And, historically, they were used in many baby foods. Under certain circumstances, these additives are valuable because they can prevent the growth of the bacterium, *Clostridium botulinum,* which causes botulism food poisoning. From the meat packers' viewpoint, nitrite offers another important advantage; it makes meat more red. With the addition of nitrite, fatty hot dogs, which would otherwise appear gray, are rendered an attractive pink color. Quite apart from appearances, however, nitrate and nitrite are highly reactive substances. Nitrates readily convert to nitrites that, in turn, combine in the stomach with chemicals called secondary amines to form nitrosamines. And nitrosamines are powerful carcinogens with a demonstrated capacity to cause cancer in most major organs of test animals.

It is only within the last few years that baby food manufacturers have removed nitrate and nitrite from their meat-containing products. They did so not as a result of FDA action, but rather as a result of pressure from public interest groups, most particularly the Washington-based Center for Science in the Public Interest. Representatives from the Center argued that botulism was not a threat because of the industry's controlled production processes; and that nitrate and nitrite were being used in baby foods essentially for cosmetic purposes. The fact that the industry ultimately withdrew the substances in the absence of government compulsion is, perhaps, the most telling evidence that commercial convenience was the motivating factor for maintaining nitrate and nitrite in baby foods.

Nitrate and nitrite are still added to vast quantities of meat regularly consumed by children (and by adults, too) — most notably frankfurters, luncheon meats, sausage, ham, and bacon — even though a convincing case for the current levels of these additives has yet to be made. What is the scope of the risk? Dr. Michael Jacobson of the Center for Science in the Public Interest has estimated a food-linked nitrosamine cancer toll ranging as high as 1000 Americans per year. And, of course, an unspecified percentage of these victims would be children.

The cancer hazards to children are not limited to childhood exposures. Carcinogenic hazards can and do arise before birth, during pregnancy — during the remarkable span of 280 days when one cell multiplies into billions of cells. New life. Traditionally, the womb has been described as a near perfect biologic space capsule. For the growing embryo, there was safety and security in the womb. We now know that this is an idealized characterization. The womb is a marvel of biologic engineering, but even this life-support system cannot completely insulate the unborn from the carcinogenic insults of the Chemical Age. Many carcinogens can traverse the placenta — the organ of communication between the fetus and the mother. Life is bound to life, and as the pregnant woman is exposed to transplacental carcinogens, so too is the developing embryo.

It is now well known that when Dr. Cesare Maltoni tested the effects of vinyl chloride gas on several hundred rats, nearly 10 percent of them developed angiosarcoma of the liver. But in addition, he found that when exposed to the gas, some of the pregnant rats subsequently produced offspring that, at birth, were afflicted with liver tumors. These newborn rats were the victims of transplacental carcinogenesis.

Perhaps one of the few saving graces of the vinyl chloride

tragedy is the fact that the production of polyvinyl chloride has historically been an all-male enterprise. Because of this mixed blessing of employment discrimination, pregnant women and their children have been spared intense workplace exposures to the cancer-causing vinyl chloride gas. But in other areas, pregnant women have been less lucky. As workers they — and the life within them — incur the cancer perils of the occupational environment. Women hold more than five and a half million of the nation's thirty million blue-collar jobs. As employment discrimination gradually eases, they are moving into jobs noted for their abnormally high cancer risk. In increasing numbers, women are becoming roofers, cement workers, and newspaper press operators. In addition, they continue to hold several hundred thousand jobs in the textile industry, where cancer hazards abound amid the dyestuffs, mists of lubricating oil, and chemically treated fabrics. Another 600,000 work in dry cleaning establishments and in shoe factories and in beauty shops — all of these workplaces harbor known chemical carcinogens. More than 120,000 women work as x-ray or laboratory technicians, seemingly clean yet carcinogenically hazardous employment. Among the millions of working women are those who stay on the job during pregnancy, many continuing to work until full term.

What is the answer to the occupational cancer risks facing mother and child alike? Except in the most extreme instances, barring pregnant women from certain jobs would prove to be a destructive policy. As Dr. Vilma Hunt of Pennsylvania State University observed, for millions of women it is not a choice of pregnancy *or* employment — "reproduction *and* work are women's lot." This being the case, there can be but one answer, an answer that will benefit all human life in the workplace: the adoption and enforcement of strict anticarcinogen safeguards throughout American industry.

The documented cancer threat to future generations is not confined to those children whose mothers, while pregnant, worked in hazardous environments. The cancer pox reaches into the womb in other ways, too. Consider the curious case of diethylstilbestrol, commonly known as DES. In 1941, Dr. Michael Shimkin and others at the National Cancer Institute reported that when they administered this synthetic hormone to mice, the males readily developed testicular tumors, and both males and females developed lymphoid tumors with disturbing frequency. Based on this laboratory evidence, Shimkin and others argued — unsuccessfully — that the FDA should disallow the use of DES as an agent for fattening beef and poultry before its sale. While the controversy concerning DES residues in meat endures right through to the 1970's, the carcinogenic hazards of DES have become evident in another, unexpected way. From the 1940's to the early 1970's, physicians prescribed DES for as many as two million pregnant women in the belief that the hormone would reduce the risk of miscarriage. Although DES proved ineffective in saving fetuses, its carcinogenic impact is now beyond dispute. DES-caused cancers are appearing not, as might be expected, in the women who had taken the hormone, but in their female children. By 1975, about 200 daughters born to mothers who had taken DES were reported to have developed vaginal cancer, some as teen-agers, others as young women. It appears that before the effects of DES run their course — some time in the next century — this transplacental carcinogen will produce cancer in the young bodies of many hundreds of female Americans.

The Chemical Age has foisted yet another carcinogenic burden upon the nation's children, both inside and outside the womb: a collection of cancer-causing pesticides. When Rachel Carson wrote *Silent Spring* in 1962, she included a chapter on the cancer dangers presented by pesticides known as chlorinated hydrocarbons. Chlorinated hydrocarbons. Molecules made up of carbon, chlorine, and hydrogen atoms. Arranged in precise chains and rings, these assorted molecular configurations have produced a steadily growing family of chemical poisons. DDT was the first of the chlorinated hydrocarbon pesticides. Acknowledging its lethal effects upon insects, Rachel Carson also discussed its impact on humans.

Dissolved in oil, as it usually is, DDT is definitely toxic. If swallowed, it is absorbed slowly through the digestive tract; it may also be absorbed through the lungs. Once it has entered the body it is stored largely in organs rich in fatty substances (because DDT itself is fat-soluble) such as the adrenals, testes, or thyroid. Relatively large amounts are deposited in the liver, kidneys, and the fat of the large, protective mesenteries that enfold the intestines.

In 1962, the evidence on DDT as a carcinogen was not yet conclusive.

In laboratory tests on animal subjects, DDT has produced suspicious liver tumors. Scientists of the Food and Drug Administration who reported the discovery of these tumors were uncertain how to classify them, but felt there was some "justification for considering them low grade hepatic cell carcinomas."

"Low grade hepatic cell carcinomas." Liver cancer. By 1969, after further animal testing, there was little room for doubt; DDT was a proven carcinogen. Finally, in 1972, it was banned, but not before virtually every American had been exposed to DDT and stored detectable quantities of the substance in the vital organs. Not only did adults accumulate DDT in their bodies; so, too, did children, including newborn infants and unborn fetuses.

But DDT was not the end of it. Other chlorinated hydrocarbon pesticides contaminated the air and food. After years of delay, in 1974 the EPA finally moved to halt the use of aldrin and dieldrin, pesticides generally applied to the nation's corn crop. During its years of maximum application, our soil and foodstuffs were absorbing between ten and twenty million pounds of aldrin and dieldrin annually. When EPA banned these pesticides, Russell Train, EPA's administrator, enunciated one of the clearest statements on record about the cancer threat to this generation — and future generations — from certain chlorinated hydrocarbon pesticides. He commented first on the extent of the biologic contamination.

It appears from recent data that virtually every individual in this country has Dieldrin stored in the body. Based on the annual national human monitoring survey conducted by this Agency, tissue samples taken during therapeutic surgery or at autopsy revealed that in 1970, 96.5 percent of all individuals tested had detectable residues of Dieldrin in their adipose tissue, with an average of 0.27 ppm. For the year 1971, 99.5 percent of all those sampled had detectable amounts that averaged 0.29 ppm.

Then Train noted dieldrin's potent cancer-causing effects.

Dieldrin-caused tumors in both mice and rats appear at a variety of sites within the body, including the liver, lungs, lymphoid tissue, thyroid, uterus and mammary glands. These tumors have resulted at highly statistically significant levels from dietary dosages as low as 0.1 ppm in the diet, which is the lowest dosage ever tested in any animal species. In short, even the lowest levels of Dieldrin produced significant cancerous effects. Furthermore, the evidence indicates that exposure to Dieldrin for periods as brief as several weeks is sufficient to cause highly significant carcinogenic effects in test animals.

Finally, Train addressed the issue of the pesticide's carcinogenicity in children.

We have now learned from a national dietary survey that young children, particularly infants from birth to one year of age, because of their high dairy product diets, consume considerably more Dieldrin on a body-weight basis than any other segment of our population. Evidence from laboratory experiments with test animals has shown that the newborn is generally more sensitive to carcinogens. Therefore, infants exposed to Dieldrin may be subjected to a considerably increased risk. It has been shown that in humans Dieldrin is transferred to the fetus during pregnancy. Thus exposure to Dieldrin begins at the earliest stages of life.

Train underscored the imminent threat to the unborn and the newborn when, just thirty days after the aldrin-dieldrin ban, he marshaled evidence against two more cancer-causing chlorinated hydrocarbon pesticides: heptachlor and chlordane, compounds widely used in American households and gardens.

Concentrations of heptachlor epoxide [a product of heptachlor or chlordane once it has been metabolized in the human body] . . . are found not only in adults, but in stillborn infants as well. The organs of 10 stillborn infants obtained in two Atlanta hospitals were found to contain an average of 0.54 ppm heptachlor epoxide. The highest levels were found in the heart, adrenal gland, and liver. The finding of residues in stillborn infants demonstrates that heptachlor epoxide is transferred from the mother to the infant across the placenta. In addition, 53 human milk samples collected in Philadelphia, and Center County, Pennsylvania, had an average concentration of heptachlor epoxide of 0.16 ppm (in milk fat) in a study reported in 1972. Three of the samples were in the 0.40 ppm to 0.49 ppm range.

These findings are disturbing since organisms that are exposed from the time of conception and then for the balance of their life are apt to be more responsive than those whose exposure begins after weaning.

Even though it is impossible . . . to assign a numerical probability to the risk that heptachlor epoxide may produce cancer in humans, some generalized conclusions are possible. The presented evidence of measurable quantitites entering man's body and further being transferred to fetuses in the uterus, indicates that humans are exposed to heptachlor epoxide from the moment of conception on throughout life. This is sufficient basis for grave concern for the possibility that humans, like the experimental mice and rats, may react to such exposure by producing malignant tumors.

No reasonable person can look at the available evidence without drawing the inference that American children — even the unborn — are subjected to carcinogenic pesticides that may kill many thousands of them before they ever reach adulthood. While direct cause-and-effect relationships are difficult to establish conclusively, epidemiologists today are seriously concerned that, in addition to other malignancies, infantile or prenatal exposure to chlorinated hydrocarbon pesticides may be associated with central nervous system tumors, including the kind that killed Jennie Day.

Even as Russell Train documented the cases against aldrin and dieldrin, and then heptachlor and chlordane, yet another chlorinated hydrocarbon, Kepone, was emerging as the latest carcinogenic pesticide. A considerable furor took place in the winter of 1975–1976 when it was disclosed that workers producing Kepone in Hopewell, Virginia, were suffering from severe poisoning. Kepone seriously damaged the brain, liver, and sperm production, leading to symptoms that included memory loss, slurred speech, twitching, nervous tremors, and sterility. Then it was learned that family members of some of the workers, particularly small children, were also displaying symptoms of Kepone poisoning, apparently the result of take-home exposures. Community anxiety was heightened further when it was revealed that the air and water for scores of miles had been contaminated with measurable levels of Kepone. The fish in the James River had become so contaminated with the pesticide that the waterway had to be closed to fishermen. As events unfolded, few citizens doubted the extreme toxicity of Kepone.

However, for the residents in and near Hopewell, the worst news may yet lie ahead. Even before the Kepone story broke, the National Cancer Institute began bioassays to determine the pesticide's cancer-causing capacity. The results released in the spring of 1976 could hardly have been more depressing. Kepone administered in high doses to male mice produced liver tumors in 88 percent of the animals; but even among the male mice tested at lower doses, 81 percent developed liver tumors. Female mice fared somewhat better. Liver tumors were found in 47 percent of those fed high doses of Kepone and in 52 percent fed lower doses.*

DDT. Aldrin. Dieldrin. Heptachlor. Chlordane. And now Kepone. The track record of chlorinated hydrocarbon pesticides is miserable and potentially calamitous. Is it unreasonable to demand a national policy that enables children to be born — as they were only twenty or thirty years ago — with livers and kidneys and brains free of cancer-causing chlorinated hydrocarbon pesticides? In 1963, President Kennedy's Science Advisory Committee on the Use of Pesticides recommended reduced reliance on chlorinated hydrocarbon pesticides, followed by their eventual elimination. Six years later, a similar recommendation was offered by the Mrak Commission (named after its chairman, Dr. Emil M. Mrak), a prestigious assembly of scientists appointed by the Secretary of HEW to study the entire question of pesticides and their relationship to environmental health. Now it is time to reopen the national debate on pesticides with an explicit

---

*This departure from the typical dose-response relationship may simply be a random aberration; or it may reflect the fact that at high doses a greater proportion of female mice succumbed to the poisonous effects of Kepone, before its carcinogenic effects were evident.

legislative proposal to ban the entire family of chlorinated hydrocarbon compounds in favor of less hazardous substitutes. The one-by-one piecemeal approach pursued by the EPA is simply inadequate. The result has been that, despite substantial evidence of their carcinogenicity, lindane, toxaphene, chlorobenzilate, mirex, and an assortment of related pesticides remain in widespread use.

To those who would argue that agricultural and economic ruin would surely follow an across-the-board ban on chlorinated hydrocarbon pesticides, the recent record belies this assertion. Since 1972, the large-scale application of DDT, aldrin, dieldrin, heptachlor and chlordane — each claimed by pesticide producers to be indispensable to the nation — has been eliminated by administrative action. Other nations have taken similar steps; some have gone further. And all of this has been accomplished with a notable absence of agricultural and economic dislocation. It now seems clear that the course of national policy will inevitably lead to an across-the-board ban on chlorinated hydrocarbon pesticides because of their demonstrated or suspected cancer-causing properties. The point is to ban them sooner rather than later.

It is bad enough that children suffer carcinogenic exposures in their first years of life, even in the womb. Now there is mounting evidence that a carcinogen's action may assure a child's cancer even *before* conception. We know that the cancerization process begins with carcinogenic damage to what were once healthy cells — perhaps cells in the lung, liver, or bladder. But what if the carcinogenic damage is inflicted upon the adult male's sperm cells? The evidence is increasingly suggestive that a carcinogen can leave an imprint on a sperm cell so that, once joined with an egg, the product of that union — the new life soon to emerge — is programmed for cancer.

In 1974, two Canadian investigators carefully reviewed the records of 386 children who died of cancer before they were five years old. In studying the records, they checked to see what kind of work the fathers of these children were engaged in at the time of their birth. They found that a disproportionately high number held jobs that exposed them to recognized cancer-causing agents: for example, service station attendants, painters, dyers, and cleaners working with solvents. There is the possibility, of course, that some of the cancer-struck children were receiving take-home exposures in infancy. But a second hypothesis advanced by the investigators is that the workplace carcinogens damaged the fathers' sperm cells, initiating a "carcinogenetic defect" that was then transmitted at conception, producing a child who subsequently was destined to develop cancer as a youngster.

This frightening hypothesis has been given added credence by evidence emerging from the vinyl chloride experience. After government researchers documented the nature and extent of the cancer epidemic among vinyl chloride workers, they began to look at related developments. They observed, for instance, that the wives of vinyl chloride workers were having miscarriages or giving birth to stillborn infants at rates far in excess of normal. Pete Gettelfinger's wife, Rita, recalled:

> Miscarriages. I had had a normal pregnancy in '51 and '52 and '53. Then Pete went to work there at [B. F. Goodrich] in 1954. I had another normal pregnancy in '56. Then I had a miscarriage in the later part of '58. I had a normal pregnancy in '60. I had a miscarriage in '62. I had a normal pregnancy in '63, and then I had another miscarriage in '65. I had three miscarriages since Pete worked there.

Several studies of the cells of vinyl chloride workers have revealed genetic damage in the form of excessive numbers of chromosomal breaks, suggesting that vinyl chloride may cause mutations in humans. Added to this are the data from a 1975 Ohio study pointing to a threefold increase in certain birth defects — central nervous system deformities — in communities exposed to vinyl chloride.

Birth defects. Chromosomal breaks. Miscarriages. Stillbirths. Containing the cancer pox is not just a matter of protecting the populace here and now; it requires an understanding that in the absence of effective policies at every level, the cancer pox is destined to become a transgenerational scourge, imposing a special burden and laying a special claim upon children for decades to come.

Part VI

Chapter 11.

Dr. Wilhelm Hueper

IN MARCH 1975, NEARLY ONE THOUSAND PEOPLE — scientists, academics, government officials, and representatives from industry and labor — gathered in New York City at a four-day Bicentennial Conference on Occupational Carcinogenesis. On the evening of the Conference's second day, there was a dinner meeting that included an award ceremony. Dr. Samuel Epstein, President of the Society for Occupational and Environmental Health, presented the Society's First Annual Award for Occupational and Environmental Honor. The recipient was Dr. Wilhelm C. Hueper (pronounced Hugh'per). Dr. Epstein began his remarks.

The Conference marks the occasion of the bicentennium of the 1775 publication by . . . Percival Pott of his classical writings on occupational cancer entitled "Chirurgical [Surgical] Observations of Cancer of the Scrotum of Chimney Sweeps."

The Society for Occupational and Environmental Health considers that this occasion is eminently suitable for us to express to you [Dr. Hueper] our deepest respects and recognition for your unique and sustained scientific contributions to occupational and environmental carcinogenesis . . . I am privileged to convey these sentiments and to present you with our first award. [But] before so doing, it would appear appropriate to presume the difficult task of capsulating and recognizing for our audience some biographic highlights and some of your pioneering contributions to humanity and to science.

Epstein then told of Dr. Hueper's medical training; of his work with the du Pont Laboratories; of his early recognition of the cancer-causing properties of radioactive materials; of his investigation and identification of carcinogenic dyestuffs. And then he described Dr. Hueper's work with the National Cancer Institute.

From 1948 to 1964 Dr. Hueper organized the . . . Laboratory of Environmental Cancer at the National Cancer Institute and established the basis for [numerous] epidemiological studies . . . His interests and research covered major fields in environmental and occupational carcinogenesis, including air and water pollution, synthetic hydrogenated coal oils, food additives, petrochemicals, and metals, including arsenic, asbestos, and chromates . . . Dr. Hueper's work clearly established recognition of the long latent period of some cancers, of the irreversibility of carcinogenic effect and of the realization that "for every cancer there is a carcinogen."

Dr. Hueper constantly stressed the social implications of his work and also . . . the need to relate problems of occupational exposures [to] problems of general environmental pollution. Dr. Hueper's work . . . [helped] establish the current consensus that most human cancer is environmental and occupational in origin and hence, preventable. Such concepts were most unpopular when Dr. Hueper first expressed them. His convictions, scientific integrity and courage gave him the strength to resist and bear with fortitude the hostility or indifference his views aroused in some quarters, particularly in government and industry . . .

Science. Industry. Government. Hueper had seen the cancer pox and fought it from each of these perspectives. As one of the truly great scientific figures of the twentieth century, he has served to demonstrate that the roots of the cancer pox are not only chemical and physical, but also economic, social, and political.

Dr. Hueper, eighty-one years old at the time of the award ceremony, could not be in New York to accept the honor. Both he and his wife were seriously ill. So arrangements had been made for Dr. Epstein to speak into a speaker-phone, and Dr. Hueper heard the concluding remarks at his home in Fort Myers, Florida.

To Wilhelm C. Hueper, M.D., Head of the Environmental Cancer Section, National Cancer Institute, Department of Health, Education and Welfare, in recognition of his role in pioneering and fostering the study of occupational and environmental cancer and in establishing the scientific and public awareness that most human cancers are caused by environmental factors and can be prevented.

As he listened over the phone, tears welled up in the old man's eyes. Along the road that had taken him from the traditional practice of pathology, to the study of cancer as an employee in private industry, and finally to sixteen stormy years with the National Cancer Institute, there had been little encouragement, but many obstacles.

Several weeks after the award ceremony, Dr. Hueper was persuaded to share his recollections of the events that shaped his career as a scientist. Speaking with an accent, and using awkwardly constructed sentences, he remembered the milestones. He remembered first the idyllic years of his youth in Germany.

I was born the second son of a middle-class family in 1894, in Schwerin, Mecklenburg, the residence of the former grand duke. For its size of 35,000 inhabitants, it had not only a beautiful environment among several lakes and large forests but offered also for the larger part of the year, performances in opera and drama and had a good museum with valuable old paintings and an extraordinary collection of fossils and stone implements. Two regiments were quartered in the city. Their bands provided additional musical entertainment. Ice skating during the winter and water sports and hiking in the woods were additional enjoyable features.

At the age of six I entered public school. Then, in 1913, I started the study of medicine as my wish had been for many years. I joined a singing fraternity in 1914.

In August 1914, the peacefulness and civility that had characterized Hueper's upbringing were abandoned to the destruction of world war. Like millions of others, this young medical student was sucked up into the holocaust. Appalled by the suffering and horror of battlefield death, the war left an indelible imprint on Hueper.

I joined as a volunteer the army although I was already at that age a sort of pacifist having read books like Nie Wieder Krieg [Never War Again] *on this subject. The next four years I spent on the French-Belgian front, first as a soldier with the infantry; then I was a medical*

aid; and, finally, I was the physician of an infantry batallion. I re-
member many times seeing there the young men that lay dead after battle.
Their bodies looked like rumpled sacks of cloth. Every one of them had a
mother somewhere. Every one of them was a mother's son!

I was taken prisoner during the first offensive of the Allied Forces and
sent to an island in the Atlantic near Bordeaux until I was sent home
after four months.

Amid what he perceived to be the pointless slaughter of
young men, Hueper's philosophy of life was forged. The pres-
ervation of life was everything. Death was the enemy. There
could be no concessions to death. And premature death — death
that could have been prevented but was not — was a concession
of criminal proportions.

Hueper completed his medical school education in 1920 and,
three years later, emigrated to the United States. During the
next six years, he was employed as a pathologist and associate
professor at the Loyola Medical School in Chicago. However, increasingly he strayed from the more traditional practice of
pathology and engaged in experimental cancer research. In
1930, he moved to the Cancer Research Laboratory of the University of Pennsylvania in Philadelphia. Once there, events were
to lead him to work for — and later break with — one of the
most powerful corporations in America, the du Pont Company.

The Cancer Research Laboratory was supported by a grant from Mr.
Irénée du Pont. This is why the atmosphere of that whole laboratory was
tilted towards chemistry. And this was really my first introduction into the
chemical aspects of cancer. The Director of the Research Laboratory was
a gynecologist, who was also the family physician of the du Pont family.
He took me sometimes along to the du Ponts' when somebody was sick. I
became introduced to them. I had lunch with them.

In 1932 I wrote to Mr. Irénée du Pont, whom I knew personally by
then. I wrote that I had come to the conclusion that the du Pont dye
workers would have the same cancer hazards to the urinary bladder as
similar workers in European plants, especially Germany, Switzerland,
and England, and that an investigation would show that these men have

an increased incidence of bladder cancer. I didn't get any personal answer to this. My boss at the Cancer Research Laboratory at the University of Pennsylvania told me several months later that the du Ponts had come to the conclusion that they had no bladder cancers among their workers. "Well," I said, "that may be, but they will get them."

Then some months later, suddenly du Pont's research director came to us in Philadelphia and said, "We have some now." I said, "How many?" And he said, "We now have twenty-three." I said, "You will have more. This is a going concern now." At that time I had already figured out that it would take about fifteen years. I told them that men who are getting cancer now are those who your company employed in 1917 when they created the dye work operation.

In 1934, the du Ponts asked Dr. Hueper to become the pathologist at its new Haskell Laboratory of Industrial Toxicology at Wilmington, Delaware. He was hired with the understanding that his special task was to "solve the puzzle" of bladder cancer in dye workers. Dr. Hueper focused first on beta-Naphthylamine and then, later, on benzidine as the suspected carcinogens. A firm believer in linking laboratory research with field study, he felt it necessary to see for himself the working conditions among du Pont's dye workers.

When I first visited the dye works for collecting exposure information, I was shown the beta-Naphthylamine operation. I talked to the foreman. It is always very important to talk with the foreman — he doesn't know why you ask the questions; the plant physicians do. You see, you need to know not only the facts but the tricks, so that you can't be fooled by anybody. I always have looked upon myself as a sort of medical detective. A medical detective must know all the tricks. So, I said to the foreman, "You have a very nice clean plant here." He said, "Oh, you should have seen it last night. We worked all night to clean it up for you."

When we were through with the visit of the beta-Naphthylamine operation, I said to the manager of the dye works, "Now I would like to see the benzidine operation." "Oh," he said, "this is not really important." I said, "I would like to see the benzidine operation now. I came this far; I would like to see it too." That was a little bit farther up the road, in a special building. When I saw that, I knew why they didn't want me there. This building they did not work all night to clean up for me. The benzidine was spread all over the place, inside and outside, on the loading platform and on the road. I said, "I know now why you did not want me to see this."

When I came back to Wilmington, I wrote a letter to the president of the company telling of the conditions, and I said that it would not help my investigation of the bladder cancer problem if they would not provide plant management that would cooperate with me. Now, the result of that letter was that I was never permitted to see the dye works again. This was my introduction to industrial ethics and professional medical integrity.

Barred from further field research, during the next several years Hueper confined his work to the laboratory, seeking to conclusively demonstrate the causal relationship between beta-Naphthylamine and the high incidence of urinary bladder cancer among du Pont workers. He finally succeeded in 1938 when he produced humanlike bladder tumors in dogs by feeding them beta-Naphthylamine. Instead of expressions of gratitude from his corporate employer, Hueper's breakthrough coincided with his dismissal by du Pont. While company officials cited economic reasons for his termination, Hueper refers to an overriding ethical dispute.

I insisted that my observations should be published. My philosophy of controlling cancer hazards in industry was fundamentally different from that of the du Pont Company. The management at that time took the view that such observations were strictly the business of the management and didn't even need to be directly communicated in all their tragic implications to the workers. My viewpoint was that as soon as the management became aware that a possible cancer hazard might exist in any of their operations, the workers should be informed why control measures were being taken so that they got the full cooperation of the men.

Although his views on corporate responsibility did not prevail, grim vindication came thirty-eight years later. Du Pont, it seems, had continued to produce beta-Naphthylamine until 1955. By its own admission, in 1976, the company revealed that 339 of 2000 workers exposed to beta-Naphthylamine from 1919 to 1955 fell victim to bladder cancer.

What Dr. Hueper had seen at du Pont — the carcinogenic filth of the work environment; what he had experienced — the barrier to his field studies; what he had concluded — that corporate officials are fully capable of regarding findings of cancer hazards as a proprietary matter that need not be shared with employees; all of this fueled his capacity for outrage. Outrage toward those who have the power and the responsibility to protect people against cancer risks, but who fail to do so.

Dr. Hueper credits his tenure at du Pont with providing "the main scientific and moral incentive" for his next undertaking, the writing of his remarkable volume *Occupational Tumors and Allied Diseases*, published in 1942. As a measure of the moral indignation he continued to harbor toward du Pont and its slogan, "Better Things for Better Living Through Chemistry," he initially proposed as the dedication to his book: "To the victims of cancer who made things for better living through chemistry." But on the advice of a friend, he amended the dedication: "This book is dedicated to the memory of those of our fellow men who have died from occupational diseases contracted while making better things for an improved living for others."

Containing both a survey of the world literature on cancer and a comprehensive catalogue of the known and suspected cancer-causing agents, Dr. Hueper's book became the scholarly weapon that he used, time and again, in a lifelong battle to encourage effective control measures to match the dangers of what he termed "the new artificial environment."

The gigantic growth of modern industry occurring in its main portion within the lifetime of men now living . . . has introduced numerous artificial, heretofore unknown, exogenous factors in constantly increasing number and variety. The creators and beneficiaries of the industrial development are thereby made potential victims of health hazards which cause numerous and diverse acute as well as chronic and insidious diseases never observed before.

Just as scientists learned in the late nineteenth century that many pathogenic micro- and macroorganisms were the environmental agents of serious infectious diseases, so too, Hueper argued, the steady increase in the incidence of cancer since 1900 was due largely to the interaction of human cells with a variety of chemical and physical agents, some of them highly carcinogenic.

More than a statement on occupational cancer, Hueper's *Occupational Tumors and Allied Diseases* stands today as a singular contribution to the modern theory of carcinogenesis. But when it was published in 1942, the book failed to attract attention commensurate with its significance. It was far ahead of current thinking about cancer. And, of course, the timing of the publication could not have been worse, coming as it did only weeks after the Japanese attack on Pearl Harbor.

The sale of the book was not impressive at all. It was a difficult time to try to interest people in the loss of life. The importance of the book — as it was finally termed a classic — appeared only after the war was over for several years. None of my books had good sales. Of course, I was disappointed at that. Naturally, anybody hopes that their books will sell. After a while, I later published books with the realization that they would draw only a limited amount of sales. I wrote them in order to put the evidence into print so that no medical director of an industrial company — no one could claim that it was not published that certain chemicals cause cancer.

For ten years, from 1938–1948, Hueper worked for the Warner Institute for Therapeutic Research, in New York. He termed the period "ten years of productive and usually harmonious scientific work in which I was permitted to conduct within reasonable limits any experimental research I selected to become engaged in." By the time he left the Warner Institute, he had rounded out his theory on the causes of cancer: occupational cancer was not an isolated phenomenon. It was the beginning of an evolving public health calamity. It was the first stage of the epidemic in slow motion.

Occupational cancer agents spread into the environment. The cancer has spread from the producers to the final commercial consumer. The same hazards spread by pollution of the environment — of the air, of the water, of the soil, of the fruit, of the cosmetics — whatever you have. As a rule, the workers get cancer first and they get it most. But the occupational hazards were only the prototypes of the environmental cancer hazards from which the total population was suffering. From the plant into the general environment.

In 1948, Dr. Hueper was offered the position of Chief of the Environmental Cancer Section of the National Cancer Institute. Then fifty-four years old, he accepted. For most men, the move would have provided an opportunity for the undisturbed pursuit of research in the twilight of a scientific career. But for Hueper, the next sixteen years were to be his most active. They were to repeatedly test his iron will, his intellectual stamina, and his sense of professional rectitude.

The Environmental Cancer Section, having only fourteen employees, was a small unit within the National Cancer Institute. Its annual budget was $90,000 in 1948 and not much more when Hueper left in 1964. Its mandate was to help identify occupational and environmental carcinogens. Dr. Hueper was well suited to this task but he saw the unit's responsibilities in much broader terms. Identification of a carcinogen was not enough. Protective measures had to be devised at once. It was unthinkable to delay — to allow people to continue to be exposed to known carcinogens and die from cancers that were preventable. These sentiments were not warmly received within the National Cancer Institute. The Institute was geared principally to research, removed from the rough and tumble of advocacy. Dr. Hueper's colleagues and his superiors preferred the quietude of research to combat over a carcinogens policy. They shied away from his blunt life-and-death characterizations. And, when pushed, they resorted to censorship as a means of containing his efforts.

When Hueper sought to explain to the Colorado Medical Society the lung cancer hazards posed to the state's uranium miners, there was no apology for the attempt to control the content of his speech.

One nice day when I submitted that manuscript for clearance, I was called later on in to the office of my director. He said, "Now, the high medical official of the Atomic Energy Committee objects against that.

They said there are quite other reasons why the uranium miners develop cancer; it's not the radioactivity. You shall omit that from your presentation." You see, the AEC was afraid that the publication of that kind of information might interfere with the continued production of atomic bombs. This is my impression, or my speculation. Anyway, I said to the director, "I will tell you something. I did not join the Public Health Service to be made a liar!"

With that, Dr. Hueper sent a copy of the uncensored manuscript to the President of the Colorado Medical Society. He, in turn, sent it to one of the Senators from Colorado, who then complained to the National Cancer Institute about the affair. These kinds of messy episodes further isolated Hueper from the National Cancer Institute establishment. Increasingly, his scientific work was subjected to the heavy hand of political interference. A "maverick," a "troublemaker" — these are the labels that he drew for his efforts. And more censorship.

In 1952, Congressman James J. Delaney (D., New York) asked Hueper to testify before his Select Committee Investigating the Use of Chemicals in Food and Cosmetics.

When I was invited by Mr. Delaney to testify before his committee, I prepared a large document — a so-called technical statement — in which I reviewed the question of additives in terms of actual and potential carcinogens in the food supply. Well, when I submitted that for clearance at NCI, I got the paper returned with the statement that since it was "unscientific" I should omit many data. I brought the paper to them again, and again they rejected it. And I submitted it again, and again they did not give it clearance. And then I said, "I will fix you." The committee became already impatient. I said, "I will fix it." I took only the introductory paragraph and the concluding paragraph and sent this silly thing in for clearance and they cleared it promptly. And the attorney for the Delaney committee, he was mad like hell, as you can imagine. He called me and I said, "This is all I can give you. These boys don't know what science is." Then officials from the National Institutes of Health suggested to me that I should refuse to testify and I said, "No, I am not refusing to testify. I am an American citizen and I have certain obligations and I am practically the only one in the United States that can really testify as an expert in those matters. I will testify and if I cannot testify as a representative of the National Cancer Institute, I will testify as a private citizen."

Dr. Hueper's testimony before the Delaney Committee was, in fact, given as a private citizen. He carefully described the cancer hazards posed by certain food additives and cosmetics in a message that he would deliver with increasing forcefulness as the years passed. Dr. Hueper was mindful of the fact that the mathematical impact of the cancer pox changed dramatically as the risks were transported beyond the occupational setting. Du Pont's beta-Naphthylamine workers had been subjected to large doses of a high-potency carcinogen, but the employee population at risk was limited in number. In contrast, when color additives with suspect cancer-causing properties are added to foods and cosmetics, virtually the entire American populace is put at risk. And, although the dosage and the carcinogenic potency of a particular color additive may be low, the population exposed is so large that the resultant cancers can ultimately number many thousands. Assume, for example, that a color additive is administered in low doses to rats and that it reliably produces only one excess tumor for every 10,000 rats tested. If this test approximates what the human experience will be (the human experience could, of course, prove far worse), then this one excess cancer for every 10,000 subjects might be expected, in time, to produce over 20,000 excess cancer cases in the American population.

It was this chilling specter of mass carcinogenesis that worried Hueper and embroiled him in the chemical additives controversy, where he was opposed by both the representatives of industry and the federal government's own Food and Drug Administration. During the early 1950's, Dr. Hueper, like others, questioned the safety of Red Dye No. 2 because of its chemical relationship to alpha-Naphthylamine and beta-Naphthylamine, two bladder carcinogens. The evidence suggested to him that the dye generates tumors in test animals. But, for Dr. Hueper, the entire controversy was symptomatic of a more fundamental failing: even if honest doubt existed as to whether this particular color additive caused cancer, he saw in its continued use a reckless abandonment of social responsibility. Hueper emphasized that Red Dye No. 2, like other color additives, is a frivolous commodity. Its use is for appearances only: to render products more saleable; to give a certain red hue to sausage and soda pop and candy and bakery goods; to make pills and medicines and cosmetics pleasant to the eye. Dr. Hueper was not opposed to color dyes per se. But where an individual dye's safety had not been convincingly demonstrated in animal tests, where there remained any suspicion about its capacity to induce cancer, his sense of social responsibility left no choice; the dye should be banned. The benefit of its continued use bore no rational relationship to the risks it posed.

Dr. Hueper was a man of conscience, not of reconciliation. His congressional testimony and his publications were matters of duty, not choice. Information was the foundation upon which protective policies must be built. Censorship was villainy. Two years after his first appearance before the Delaney Committee, he submitted another paper reviewing the problem of carcinogens in food and other consumer goods. Clearance was refused on this paper, too, with the allegation that it contained scientifically unjustified claims. A man of inordinate persistence, Dr. Hueper pursued the matter to the point of having Congressman John Moss of California write a letter to HEW inquiring whether the doctor's publications were being censored. Despite denials, Hueper later confirmed that he was not only the victim of censorship, but the victim of government–industry collusion as well.

At a meeting in the later 1950's in New Jersey, I was informed during an informal conversation with a former member of the Haskell Laboratory that he had read for the du Pont management many of my manuscripts which I had submitted to the editorial board of NCI for comments. Someone in the Public Health Service found it expedient to engage in this unethical collusion and potential sabotage of governmental cancer research paid for by American taxpayers. When I protested in a memorandum against such peculiar cooperation between government and industrial management, I met a wall of silence. Nobody seemed to know who might be responsible for this knavery.

Over the years, Hueper became something of a specialist in drawing attention to his memoranda. Frequently, he would skip links in the Public Health Service's chain of command and send his memos directly to the Secretary of HEW, a practice sure to irritate even the most self-confident administrator. Dr. Rod Heller was Director of the National Cancer Institute during this period, and Hueper recalls his reaction.

Heller once called my attention to [my memoranda sent directly to the Secretary] *and said he didn't like it and I should send all the memoranda first to him. I said, "Yes, I can sympathize with your attitude, but I know that you would condemn some of my memoranda to the waste-basket. And for that reason I want to have them known on top. And this is the reason why I have chosen this way of communicating my knowledge to the Secretary of the Department and sending you only a copy and the Surgeon General only a copy. And to be sure that the Secretary would get the letter first, I sent you the copy two days later." They didn't like that kind of tactic, and I understand that.*

His detractors described him as "abrasive," "teutonic," and "uncompromising." Hueper could be all of those things. But above all he was a superb scientist. The sheer breadth of his knowledge about carcinogenesis was unmatched. Heller appreciated his expertise and, to his credit, defended Hueper against those who wanted to see him fired. Dr. Hueper managed to stay on, but the price of tenure was high. When he joined the National Cancer Institute in 1948, it was understood that there were to be two aspects to his work. One aspect was experimental carcinogenesis: testing substances on animals to determine their cancer-causing properties. The second aspect was epidemiology: conducting field studies to determine the cancer-causing consequences to workers and other population groups exposed to recognized or suspected carcinogens. Epidemiology could be politically explosive work. It meant going into plants and surveying working conditions. It meant reviewing plant records. It meant reviewing death records. In its totality, cancer epidemiology was a matter of unearthing skeletons: in the uranium industry, in the dyestuffs industry, in the chromate industry. It invariably raised ugly questions of responsibility and legal liability for occupational and community cancer deaths. Reminiscent of his experience at du Pont fourteen years earlier, in 1952 the order came down through channels: Dr. Hueper was forbidden to do his epidemiologic work. A quarter of a century later, although physically frail, Dr. Hueper still bellows with rage as he recounts the event.

I was forbidden to contact state health departments and industrial concerns. They restricted me to do only experimental laboratory work. But my main interest was the human beings. I am not fundamentally interested in mice! I am interested in men! This is the reason why I came to the Public Health Service. I didn't want to produce another variety of mouse cancer. I wanted to save the human population from this incredible misery of cancer. When I was in Philadelphia and I was the pathologist of a cancer hospital, I saw all that at close sight. Then later on I saw all that misery of the bladder cancer — most of them at that time died. I never lost that. My main interest was the human misery. That goes for all my writings. I don't care how many mice die of cancer! That was a minor matter to me! But I didn't want to see that human beings should die from cancer when that was avoidable.

Hueper had no illusions about the motivation for the restrictive order.

My work led to political difficulties. It is easy to work on genetics or viruses or on biochemistry. There are no implications whatever. And there are no political difficulties. My work led to political difficulties with Congress and with individual commercial parties. My work directly confronted them with the problems of what substances cause cancer. I was highly controversial, and politicians preferred to ignore the important issues my work was advancing.

Ironically, some of Hueper's most enduring contributions can be traced to the limits placed upon his activities. Blocked from engaging in laborious field studies, he turned increasingly to other pursuits. A prolific writer, he continued to publish at an astounding pace notwithstanding the recurrent problems of censorship. Today, five major books and more than 350 publications bear his name. Just a few of the titles substantiate the encyclopedic nature of his knowledge of cancer causation: "Air Pollution and Cancer of the Lung" (1953), "Experimental Cancers in Rats Produced by Chromium Compounds" (1959), "Cancer Hazards from Natural and Artificial Water Pollutants" (1960), "Chemically Induced Skin Cancers in Man" (1963), "Toxic and Carcinogenic Hazards to the Human Population from Pesticides and Pesticide Residues" (1963).

Dr. Hueper was one of the few scientists to write about carcinogenic contaminants in cosmetics, an area of study that, to this day, has been badly neglected by both researchers and policymakers. In both his articles and his books, he cautioned against the potential cancer hazards — breast cancer and uterine cancer — associated with the use of estrogens in cosmetic preparations. And, he warned against the unregulated use of certain hair dyes, lip waxes, and coal tars, citing the dangers of skin cancer, cancer of the lip, and liver and bladder cancers.

Beyond his writings, in his final years with the National Cancer Institute, Hueper undertook to build an international scientific consensus on the environmental origins of cancer. In 1956, he traveled to Rome, where the International Union Against Cancer assembled a panel of scientific authorities from throughout the world to discuss potential cancer hazards posed by chemical additives and contaminants in food. Recognizing what it termed "the urgent necessity for international collaboration for the protection of mankind," the scientists unanimously adopted a series of resolutions dealing with the carcinogenic dangers of a number of color additives, preservatives, pesticides, and hormones administered to livestock — all increasingly contaminating the food supply. So persuasive was the work of the Rome conference that, in 1958, Congressman Delaney and others cited the scientists' recommendations as the principal reason for seeking new legislative controls on food additives.

Finally, in the fall of 1963, just a year before his retirement,

Dr. Hueper joined with eleven of his colleagues in Geneva, at a meeting of the World Health Organization Expert Committee on the Prevention of Cancer. The committee's study, later embodied in a famous report, *Prevention of Cancer*, marked a new beginning in efforts to draw attention to the need for preventive cancer policies. The committee noted that the emphasis on cancer prevention had historically been limited to early diagnosis of the disease, with too little attention given to the accumulating knowledge regarding environmental carcinogens implicated in the causation of human cancer. The committee asserted:

The potential scope of cancer prevention is limited by the proportion of human cancers in which extrinsic factors are responsible. These include all environmental carcinogens (whether already identified or not) as well as "modifying factors" that favour [tumor formation] of apparently intrinsic origin (e.g., hormonal imbalances, dietary deficiencies, and metabolic defects). The types of cancer that are thus influenced, directly or indirectly, by extrinsic factors include many tumours of the skin and mouth, the respiratory, gastro-intestinal and urinary tracts, hormone-dependent organs (such as the breast, thyroid and uterus) and haematopoietic and lymphopoietic systems — which, collectively, account for more than three-quarters of human cancer. It would seem, therefore, that the majority of human cancer is potentially preventable.

"It would seem, therefore, that the majority of human cancer is potentially preventable." When this draft language was approved by the committee at its concluding session, Professor L. M. Shabad, an eminent cancer researcher from the USSR Academy of Medical Sciences, leaned over to Dr. Hueper and asked, "Isn't it a great source of satisfaction to you that the committee has come to this conclusion?" Hueper replied, "Yes, it is indeed." But Dr. Hueper knew from experience that the distance between scientific understanding and effective public policy can stretch half a lifetime — or more.

Chapter 12.

Toward a New Ethic

In 1964, Dr. Hueper turned seventy, the age of mandatory retirement from federal service. His mind alert, his health good, he used the next five years to complete work on three books that were to become a classical trilogy: *Chemical Carcinogenesis and Cancers* (1964), *Occupational and Environmental Cancers of the Respiratory Tract* (1967), and *Occupational and Environmental Cancers of the Urinary System* (1969). The three books, totaling more than 1300 pages, constituted a detailed summary of the scientific evidence that pinpointed the occupational and environmental origins of most human cancers; the books also provided a carefully considered blueprint for the adoption of effective policies to reduce occupational and environmental cancer hazards and, thereby, ultimately reduce the toll of human cancer. It is against this blueprint for protective policies that the neglect of recent years must be measured.

The screening and pretesting of chemicals formed the baseline of Dr. Hueper's blueprint. Without carcinogenesis bioassays — without systematic testing on laboratory animals — many existing cancer hazards would remain undetected, and new chemicals would continue to be introduced into the economy without our foreknowledge of their cancer-causing properties. Despite the obvious need for this kind of thorough assessment, Congress let the years pass — and the dangers mount — before finally adopting the necessary legislation.

Beyond the imperative of carcinogenesis bioassays, Dr. Hueper's blueprint recognized that carcinogens fall into one of two principal categories. The first category includes what are termed natural carcinogens, such as the sun's ultraviolet radiation or the arsenic washed down from the mountains. Little or nothing could be done about the sources of these carcinogenic exposures. But, fortunately, these naturally occurring carcinogens represent a relatively minor proportion of the total carcinogenic burden. It is the second category of carcinogens — the man-made carcinogens — that represent the far larger threat to the human species. And here, Dr. Hueper stressed that a great deal could be done. A number of these man-made carcinogens can, and should, be banned by law. Regrettably, this straightforward approach has rarely become national policy. Benzidine, for example, was long ago demonstrated to be a potent source of bladder cancer among dye workers. Several Western European countries and Japan simply outlawed its manufacture and use. These governments recognize that the economic importance of benzidine is so far outweighed by the cancer risks that it presents, that reason compels its outright elimination from the environment. In contrast, the United States maintains the dubious distinction of being the industrial world's principal hold-out on benzidine. United States policy continues to sacrifice hundreds of human lives, not only among exposed workers, but also among high school and college students, who study in chemistry laboratories where benzidine is used with little apparent regard for its cancer-causing properties.

As for those man-made carcinogens that are not banned by law, Dr. Hueper stressed the need for the strictest regulatory controls. Standards should be established to reduce exposure to the minimum level technologically possible. Of course, strict standards assume the *existence* of standards. This is an unwarranted assumption in the context of current United States policy. Many recognized and suspected cancer-causing agents — carbon tetrachloride, chloroform, wood dust, trichloroethylene — are not yet subject to nationally established carcinogens standards. Even agents that were identified one hundred or two hundred years ago as potent carcinogens — arsenic, and coal soots and coal tars — have gone unregulated, delayed most recently by Gerald Ford's presidential order requiring inflation-impact statements prior to regulatory action.

Dr. Hueper urged, as others have since, that a permit or

licensing system be instituted to require proof of all appropriate safeguards *before* a cancer-causing substance could be manufactured or used. There should be no misunderstanding about the fact that a properly operating permit system will lead to a shutdown of some of the filthiest and most dangerous factories and businesses. This was the recent experience in Pennsylvania, when that state adopted a permit system covering a series of recognized carcinogens, including beta-Naphthylamine, the same substance that Dr. Hueper implicated in the bladder cancer epidemic that struck du Pont's workers. Among the Pennsylvania firms affected by the law, most simply ceased producing beta-Naphthylamine. But Pennsylvania's law could only extend to the state border, and in 1973, federal officials investigating a plant in Georgia were dismayed to find workers sloshing in slurry tanks hip deep in beta-Naphthylamine. This single experience can be interpreted in one of two ways: with despair, as one more illustration that law is a limited tool for shaping human conduct; or, as a hopeful sign that laws do indeed affect human conduct. The Pennsylvania permit system worked — and worked well; the failure was jurisdictional, not conceptual. If there had been a *national* permit system instead of an uneven state-by-state policy, the protection of the law would not have been confined to Pennsylvania; it would have extended to every workplace across the country.

Of course, Dr. Hueper's blueprint went beyond the occupational context. His plan called for the establishment and enforcement of new environmental laws to halt carcinogenic contamination of the nation's air, soil, food, and medical supplies. He envisioned an important role for the criminal law in curbing cancer hazards; his writings included impassioned pleas for the adoption and application of criminal sanctions where violations of law exposed others to the perils of known carcinogens.

Human society must assume responsibility for assuring its own ordered and moral existence . . . protecting without distinction and compromise the health and welfare of all its members. A reckless, callous and irresponsible exposure of . . . [others] to avoidable and unnecessary cancer hazards for obtaining special financial gain by private parties obviously violates the legitimate interest which the human society must assume in such matters. The mere payment of monetary compensation to the individual suffering from the results of such practices is scarcely an adequate judgment and deterrent. Such violations of basic human rights should not be condoned under the pretext that they cannot be abolished without creating undue economic hardship to the violating parties and without hindering necessary economic progress, since the present laws do not extend to any private person and organization a license for making an arbitrary decision [as to] who may be maimed and who is expendable, without rendering an accounting for such acts.

Many have died because of "reckless, callous and irresponsible exposure . . . to avoidable and unnecessary cancer hazards," but those responsible have not been prosecuted and jailed for their deadly conduct. There is a twofold purpose for the establishment and effective enforcement of criminal laws. In the first instance, these laws serve as an instrument of justice in punishing wrongdoers; and second, they serve to deter others from similar antisocial acts. To date, there has been neither justice nor deterrence in dealing with those identifiable individuals who are responsible, in part, for the cancer pox.

In creating a blueprint for an effective cancer prevention policy, Dr. Hueper was cognizant of the fact that the cancer pox is largely reflective of governmental institutions that are inadequate to the challenge of the Chemical Age. The solution, he believed, must involve the creation of institutional power strong enough to offset and reverse the impetus toward the cancer pox. During his years at the National Cancer Institute, Dr. Hueper proposed and argued for the organization of a separate Environmental Cancer Institute. In addition to epidemiologic and experimental study of environmental cancer hazards, the proposed new institute would actively promote a variety of control measures in the medicolegal and legislative areas. It was a proposal that had merit when he first advanced it two decades ago; and, now, in the aftermath of another twenty years of cancer policy failures, the proposal takes on an urgency bordering on desperation.

The chief problem in the evolution of a national cancer policy has been the inability to find a place for cancer specialists like

Hueper — scientists and others who are not simply technicians but who are also enthusiastic advocates for policies protective of the public's health. Historically, these individuals have been scattered throughout numerous federal agencies, each having only partial responsibility for controlling carcinogenic hazards. Like Dr. Hueper, many scientists have been buried in the catacombs of the National Cancer Institute, a research agency in which advocacy is frowned upon because it invariably renders the Institute "offensive" to powerful economic and political interests.

What is needed is a new Cancer Prevention Agency that, unlike OSHA, the EPA, or the FDA, would have no regulatory responsibility of its own. Unlike these other agencies, it would not have to develop standards and regulations that seek to "balance" commercial interests against health considerations. Instead, its mission would be to offer an institutional voice on behalf of the public's health — and nothing else. Its mandate would be advocacy, advocacy of cancer prevention measures before the disparate agencies that currently share responsibility for cancer policy:

• Advocacy. Advocacy at OSHA hearings to press for the adoption of additional standards controlling occupational carcinogens and to strengthen those few standards already adopted.

• Advocacy at EPA hearings to secure the adoption and enforcement of regulations to safeguard the air, water, and land from the industrial dumping of carcinogens.

• Advocacy before the FDA to demand far greater vigilance so that the FDA will never again wait for more than twenty years before it even begins to act against carcinogenic contaminants like DES and Red Dye No. 2.

In addition to testimony before these regulatory agencies, the proposed Cancer Prevention Agency should be empowered to challenge the inadequacy of agency regulations in the courts. And its mandate should also include responsibility for carrying the cancer prevention message to Congress in order to secure the increased budget appropriations necessary for effective cancer prevention policies: a greater budget for OSHA to hire thousands of new compliance officers; a greater budget for NIOSH to conduct scores of occupational cancer field studies; a greater budget for the EPA to develop and enforce anticarcinogen environmental regulations.

Consider for a moment the misplaced emphasis in current cancer policy. It is generally recognized that perhaps 90 percent of all human cancer is environmental in origin. Yet, even by the most generous estimates, less than 20 percent of the nearly $1 billion annually budgeted for the National Cancer Institute is channeled toward prevention. In addition, when there is an accounting of all of the funds actually spent by all of the federal regulatory agencies in regulating known carcinogens, it turns out that less than $300 million annually is directed to these vital efforts.

An advocacy-oriented Cancer Prevention Agency could change these priorities. But it could do still more. It could serve as an activist force in promoting new legislation essential to a humanistic cancer control policy. For example, the agency could lobby for legislation to overhaul worker compensation laws, enabling more workers and their families to at least recover monetary damages for job-caused cancers. It could also lobby for anticigarette legislation, including the removal of tax subsidies for tobacco and the establishment of an anticigarette media campaign.

The Cancer Prevention Agency could also be expected to generate innovative methods to foster tough anticancer policies. For example, just as environmental-impact statements and inflation-impact statements are now required to accompany major regulatory decisions, the Cancer Prevention Agency could regularly develop mortality-impact statements. These statements would be reasoned estimates of the number of lives likely to be lost to cancer depending upon the laxity or stringency of federal policies regarding a specific occupational or environmental carcinogen. As difficult and as painful as this task might be, it is essential that those who promulgate regulations that seek to balance economic interests against health interests begin to confront — in writing — the range of possible cancer deaths associated with specific policy decisions.

The proposed Cancer Prevention Agency need not be large. A relatively small group of scientists, technicians, and lawyers —

perhaps no more than 100 individuals, but all advocates — could have a major impact in redirecting national cancer policy along more productive lines. To be effective, however, the agency must be independent of the National Cancer Institute and all other existing agencies. And its funding must be guaranteed by a statutory formula, so that its advocacy will not be tempered by the threat of debilitating budget cutbacks.

The proposed Cancer Prevention Agency is only a starting point. It must not be looked upon as an end in itself; rather, it should be regarded as an institutional vehicle capable of harnessing a national anticancer constituency that now has no effective representation within the federal government. But neither the Cancer Prevention Agency nor protective cancer policies will come to pass unless a still larger failure is remedied: the failure of political leadership to popularize cancer prevention as an operative philosophy. Upon reflection, this failure of political leadership is not surprising; preventive policies entail special problems requiring uncommon, even courageous leadership. One of the principal problems of prevention is that it is without glamor and without drama. If a surgeon transplants a human heart, the whole world applauds. But if 1000 heart attacks are avoided by a community program to take blood pressure readings so that those found to be at risk can be treated, there is no applause at all. On a national scale, we recently witnessed this same phenomenon when the automobile speed limit was reduced to 55 miles per hour as an energy conservation measure. Approximately 10,000 lives have been saved annually because of this change in policy, but there are no cheers. There is no collective expression of national gratitude. Prevention rarely produces any heroes in the traditional sense because those whose lives are spared by preventive policies remain forever anonymous. That is the nature of prevention. It is tragedy averted. It is an act of logic and compassion. It is an act of utmost social responsibility. But it is not a dramatic endeavor.

In the case of cancer prevention, the problem is particularly aggravated. An infectious epidemic, such as influenza, spans a relatively short period of time. In a matter of weeks, the disease first appears in the population; then it strikes increasing numbers of victims; it peaks; and then it subsides. In contrast, the cancer pox — Dr. Hueper's epidemic in slow motion — is an epidemic stretching over decades. The long latent period between exposure to a carcinogen and the resultant cancer lulls us into a false sense of well-being. Prevention in this context is a doubly difficult matter because, for most carcinogens, even the most stringent protective measures taken today will not yield a demonstrable improvement in cancer incidence and mortality trends for ten years or more. To a can-do society accustomed to quick results, this is a bitter and depressing message.

The challenge, then, is not to score a dramatic early victory over the cancer pox. That is not a realistic prospect. The decades of neglect in controlling carcinogenic exposures have assured a worsening mortality rate — perhaps a sharply worsening mortality rate — in the years immediately ahead. The challenge is to rapidly and significantly reduce the total carcinogenic burden — the cumulative load of occupational and environmental carcinogens borne by the populace. If this can be done, and it can, the cancer pox will be slowed during the next ten to fifteen years, and, with continued vigilance, the annual toll of cancer victims might actually begin to decline by the end of the century.

Dr. Hueper has estimated that if effective preventive measures were instituted without further delay, the reduction in the total carcinogenic burden could be expected, in time, to lead to a 50 percent overall improvement in cancer incidence. Other estimates recently developed at the National Cancer Institute appear to corroborate Hueper's projection as an achievable goal. What is lacking is the leadership essential to success in this social enterprise. It will require the most extraordinary political leadership to educate the public and other politicians to the need for adopting preventive policies today that will not begin to bring about the decline of the cancer epidemic until the year 1990 or 1995, or even until the early part of the twenty-first century. An undertaking of this character requires elected officials with a vision extending beyond the next election or the next three or four or five elections. It calls for the kind of leadership so far too scarce in the Congress, in the regulatory agencies, and in the presidency itself.

When he was in charge of the Carcinogenesis Program of the National Cancer Institute, Dr. Umberto Saffiotti described cancer as having the qualities of a social disease. It is a disease that is largely the product of the way in which we have structured and managed — or mismanaged — a modern industrial nation. With no miraculous medical solutions in sight, there is no alternative but to address this social disease with social solutions. Some of these social solutions will include: the pretesting of chemicals; the licensing of all commercial producers and users of carcinogens; and the imposition of the strictest protective regulations coupled with no-nonsense enforcement. Further social solutions will involve public education: to underscore the risks of smoking, excessive drinking, too much exposure to sunlight, or unwise dietary habits.

But still more is required. The deans who head the nation's public and private medical schools must adopt the view that an understanding of the fundamental aspects of cancer prevention is essential to a modern medical school curriculum. They must recognize that a medical education is inadequate if it lacks a thorough grounding in the principles and techniques for identifying and avoiding unnecessary cancer risks.

The men and women who head the nation's communications network — officials from radio, television, and the print media — have a similar responsibility. It is not enough to report the individual cancer calamities as they occur: vinyl chloride, DES, Premarin. The impression conveyed to the ordinary citizen is that these are isolated tragedies that can be dismissed as unrelated to one another. But it is precisely the relationship of these events — the fact that they are the separate components of a long-term cancer epidemic — that must not be lost. Editors and news directors have a special obligation to see to it that the reporting of current cancer tragedies is supplemented by larger, in-depth features that do not hesitate to criticize failures in public policy. This requires a commitment of journalistic resources — time, money, and personnel — far in excess of what has been invested to date.

Political, educational, and journalistic leadership is not easy to come by. On occasion, society is exceptionally fortunate to be blessed with the spontaneous emergence of able leaders. But more often than not, leadership springs from broad-based citizen discontent. It is in this connection that individual and collective citizen action bears upon the future direction of the cancer pox. The citizenry's steady insistence upon answers to probing questions is an effective means of advancing protective policies. Those who hold positions of high authority in government, in business, and in labor must be confronted with an unremitting series of inquiries: What is your attitude toward cancer prevention policy? What are the specific elements of your program for cancer prevention? To what extent are you prepared to commit public and private expenditures to this effort? What are you actually *doing* to lessen exposure to known and suspected carcinogens — at the workplace, in the general environment, in the channels of commerce?

All of this really constitutes a new ethic in which prevention becomes the centerpiece of national cancer policy. The idea of the prevention ethic is not to eliminate all cancer risks; that is not possible. Nor is it to render life a fearsome experience fixated on death from cancer. Instead, the idea is to take those reasonable steps that will significantly reduce the threat of cancer, so that, in the aggregate, a greater percentage of people will live out their lives free of the misery and suffering that cancer now brings to so many.

This is what Dr. Hueper had in mind when, his own life drawing to a close, he looked to the future with a note of measured optimism:

We must try to do the best for mankind — to keep people healthy and to keep them alive. We can have a better future than the past. I am sure that we will not produce paradise, and I am sure that we will still have cancer with us. But if we do what we should, we will have at least made a beginning toward the reasonable, sensible, and effective prevention of cancer. That is my testament.

Notes and Sources

Preface

Page x–"Time often measurable in years." Schmeck, Harold M., Jr. "Report on Cancer Hopeful on Gains, but Predicts No Sudden Cure," *New York Times*, November 1, 1974, p. 14.

Page xi–have remained almost unchanged. Greenberg, Daniel S. "Cancer: Now, the Bad News," *Washington Post*, January 19, 1975, pp. C1 and C4; U.S., Department of Health, Education and Welfare, *End Results in Cancer*, edited by Lillian M. Axtel (NIH 73-272), 1972.

Page xi–It accounts for just 1 percent. *'75 Cancer Facts and Figures*. New York: American Cancer Society, 1974, p. 5.

Page xi–survival rates are still tragically low. Cutler, Sidney J., et al. "Trends in Survival Rates of Patients with Cancer," *New England Journal of Medicine* (July 17, 1975): 122–124.

Page xii–recognize the chemical origins of cancer. Hueper, Wilhelm C. *Occupational Tumors and Allied Diseases*. Springfield, Ill.: Thomas, 1942.

Page xii–these are the causative agents. Hueper, Wilhelm C., and Conway, W. D. *Chemical Carcinogenesis and Cancers*. Springfield, Ill.: Thomas, 1964, pp. 19–39.

Page xii–the vast majority of all human cancers. U.S., Department of Health, Education and Welfare, *Report of Carcinogenesis Program, Fiscal Year 1975*, Division of Cancer Cause and Prevention, National Institutes of Health (NIH 76-991), p. 1; World Health Organization, *Prevention of Cancer*, Report of a WHO Expert Committee (WHO Technical Report Series No. 276), 1964, p. 4; Chriss, Nicholas C. "Human Exposure to Chemicals Suspected in 80% of Cancers," *Los Angeles Times*, March 31, 1974, Part I, pp. 1 and 17.

Page xiii–perhaps up to 90 percent. Epstein, Samuel S. "Environmental Determinants of Human Cancer," *Cancer Research* 34 (1974); 2425–2435; *The Sixth Annual Report of the Council on Environmental Quality*, Council on Environmental Quality, December, 1975, pp. 1–41; Higginson, John. "Present Trends in Cancer Epidemiology," in *Proceedings of the Eighth Canadian Cancer Research Conference*, edited by J. F. Morgan. Canadian Cancer Conference, vol. 8, Oxford: Pergamon Press, 1969, pp. 40–75.

Page xiii–over 370,000 Americans. *'76 Cancer Facts and Figures*. New York: American Cancer Society, 1975, p. 9.

Page xiii–These statistics reflect more than. U.S. Department of Health, Education and Welfare, *Mortality Trends for Leading Causes of*

Death: United States — 1950-69, Vital and Health Statistics, series 20, no. 16, National Center for Health Statistics (HRA 74-1852), March, 1974, pp. 11–18; U.S. Department of Health, Education and Welfare, *Monthly Vital Statistics Report: Advance Report Final Mortality Statistics, 1974*, National Center for Health Statistics (HRA 76-1120), vol. 24, no. 11, supplement, February 3, 1976, p. 2.

Page xiii–cancer is on the rise . . . children. Michael, Paul. *Tumors of Infancy and Childhood*. Philadelphia: Lippincott, 1964, pp. 1–7.

Page xiii–nearly one of every five Americans who died. *'75 Cancer Facts and Figures*, p. 3.

Chapter 1 Joseph Fitman

Pages 3–18 Author's interviews with Joseph and Virginia Fitman.

Chapter 2 Job-Caused Cancer

Page 20–high-risk occupational cancer environment. Hueper, Wilhelm C., and Conway, W. D. *Chemical Carcinogenesis and Cancers*. Springfield, Ill.: Thomas, 1964, p. 35; World Health Organization. *IARC Monographs on the Evaluation of Carcinogenic Risk of Chemicals to Man, vol. 1*, International Agency for Research on Cancer, 1972, pp. 29–36.

Page 20–the University of Pittsburgh undertook a massive study. Redmond, Carol K., and Breslin, Patricia P. "Comparison of Methods for Assessing Occupational Hazards," *Journal of Occupational Medicine*, 17 (May 1975): 313–317.

Page 21–fiber-glass particles that are now suspect as a cancer-causing agent. U.S. Department of Health, Education and Welfare, Dement, John M. "Environmental Aspects of Fibrous Glass Production," Division of Field Studies and Clinical Investigations, National Institute for Occupational Safety and Health; U.S. Department of Health, Education and Welfare, Bayliss, David L., and Wagoner, Joseph K. "Mortality Patterns Among Fibrous Glass Production Workers," (Preliminary Report) Division of Field Studies and Clinical Investigations, National Institute for Occupational Safety and Health.

Page 21–is a suspect carcinogen. Hueper, *Chemical Carcinogenesis*, pp. 21 and 29.

Page 22–"one of the wonders of the living world." Carson, Rachel. *Silent Spring*. Boston, Massachusetts: Houghton Mifflin, 1962.

Page 22–the site of a cancer is largely dependent upon the nature of the carcinogen. Hueper, *Chemical Carcinogenesis*.

Pages 23–24 896 page text. Hueper, Wilhelm C. *Occupational Tumors and Allied Diseases*. Springfield, Ill.: Thomas, 1942.

Page 24–Rubber workers are dying of cancer at rates from 50

percent to 300 percent greater than general population. McMichael, A. J., et al., "Solvent Exposure and Leukemia Among Rubber Workers: An Epidemiologic Study," *Journal of Occupational Medicine* 17 (April 1975): 234–239.

Page 24–Steelworkers are most vulnerable to coal tar emissions. Lloyd. J. William. "Long-Term Mortality Study of Steelworkers (Part) V. Respiratory Cancer in Coke Plant Workers," *Journal of Occupational Medicine* 13 (February 1971): 53–68.

Page 25–Asbestos workers die from lung cancer at a rate more than seven times that of comparable control groups. Selikoff, Irving J., et al. "Cancer Risk of Insulation Workers in the United States," in *Biological Effects of Asbestos*, monograph no. 8, International Agency for Research on Cancer, 1974, pp. 209–216.

Page 25–Mesothelioma has become a relatively commonplace cause of death. Brodeur, Paul. "Reporter At Large: The Magic Mineral," *The New Yorker*, October 12, 1968, pp. 117–165.

Page 25–notoriously high rates of urinary bladder cancer. Hueper, *Chemical Carcinogenesis*.

Page 25–94 percent later developed bladder tumors. Saffiotti, Umberto. "The Laboratory Approach to the Identification of Environmental Carcinogens," in *Proceedings of the Ninth Canadian Cancer Research Conference*, edited by P. G. Scholefield, vol. 9, Toronto: University of Toronto Press, 1972, p. 26.

Page 25–lung cancer rate is astonishing, upwards of 50 percent of all deaths. Hueper, Wilhelm C. "Environmental Cancer Hazards," *Journal of Occupational Medicine* 14 (February 1972): 149–153.

Page 25–two million workers are exposed to the solvent benzene. U.S. Department of Health, Education and Welfare, *Criteria for a Recommended Standard: Occupational Exposure to Benzene*, NIOSH.

Page 25–1.5 million laborers are exposed to inorganic arsenic. *Criteria for a Recommended Standard*: Occupational Exposure to Inorganic Arsenic, NIOSH.

Page 25–an ever-expanding list of workers who hold jobs posing special cancer risks. Author's communications with NIOSH officials.

Page 28–Hueper, Wilhelm C. speech entitled "Organized Labor and Occupational Cancer Hazards," prepared for delivery before the Executive Council of the AFL-CIO, 1959.

Page 29–annual budget of the national cancer program. U.S. Department of Health, Education and Welfare, *The Strategic Plan*, National Cancer Program (NIH 74-569), January 1973, chap. 5, pp. 1–10.

Pages 30–31 Brodeur, "The Magic Mineral."

Page 30–Millions of workers are in intimate occupational contact with asbestos. Letter to James D. Hodgson, Secretary of Labor, from

George H. R. Taylor, Executive Secretary, AFL-CIO Standing Committee on Safety and Occupational Health, November 4, 1971.

Pages 30–31 Selikoff, Irving J., et al. "Asbestos Exposure and Neoplasia," *Journal of the American Medical Association* 188 (1964): 22–26.

Page 31–Selikoff, Irving J., et al. "Asbestos Exposure, Smoking and Neoplasia," *Journal of the American Medical Association* 204 (1968): 106–112.

Page 31–a victim of pleural mesothelioma. Author's communications with attorney Joseph Miller, workers' compensation specialist, Los Angeles.

Page 32–Dr. Selikoff and the time bomb effect of decades-old asbestos exposures. "Asbestos Union Keeps Grim Watch for Cancer," Labor Occupational Health Program, *Monitor*, vol. 2 (November-December 1975): 2.

Page 32–Selikoff and labor union leaders urged adoption of standard. "Occupational Safety and Health Standards: Standard for Exposure to Asbestos Dust," *Federal Register* 37 (June 7, 1972): 11318–11322.

Page 33–*Evaluation of Environmental Carcinogens: Report to the Surgeon General, USPHS by the Ad Hoc Committee on the Evaluation of Low Levels of Environmental Chemical Carcinogens*, April 22, 1970.

Page 35–Rohm and Haas. Hricko, Andrea. "Slow Death in the Workplace," *The Progressive* March 1975, pp. 28–29.

Page 35–Diamond Shamrock Chemical Company. U.S. Department of Health, Education and Welfare, "Field Survey: Diamond Shamrock Chemical Company," Division of Field Studies and Clinical Investigations, National Institute for Occupational Safety and Health, 1972.

Page 36–BCME may be present in a wide range of industrial processes. U.S. Department of Health, Education and Welfare, "Hazard Review of Bis(chloromethyl)ether (BCME)," prepared by Donald V. Lassiter, Office of Research and Standards Development, National Institute for Occupational Safety and Health, June, 1973.

Page 36–OSHA issued its standards. "Occupational Safety and Health Standards: Carcinogens," *Federal Register* 39 (January 29, 1974): 3756–3797.

Page 38–OSHA's annual budget. Address of Congressman David R. Obey (D., Wis.) before the Society for Occupational and Environmental Health, Washington, D.C., December, 1974.

Page 39–"as if evil is its own reward." Brodeur, Paul. "Annals of Industry — V," *The New Yorker*, November 26, 1973, p. 174.

Page 39–George C. Guenther and his confidential memo to Department of Labor. "The Watergate Memo," *Facts & Analysis: Occupational Health and Safety*, Industrial Union Department, AFL-CIO, vol. 18, July 22, 1974.

Chapter 3 Pete Gettelfinger

Pages 43–55 Author's interviews with Pete and Rita Gettelfinger, and one of their children, Janice.

Page 44–Vinyl chloride was first produced. "Occupational Safety and Health Standards: Standard for Exposure to Vinyl Chloride," *Federal Register* 39 (October 4, 1974): 35890–35898.

Page 44–In March 1973, Dr. Creech learned of a case of angiosarcoma. Creech, J. L., Jr., and Johnson, M. N. "Angiosarcoma of the Liver in the Manufacture of Polyvinyl Chloride," *Journal of Occupational Medicine* 16 (March, 1974): 150–151.

Page 46–Cancers that begin in the liver account for about 1 in 40 of all malignancies. Robbins, Stanley L. *Pathology.* 3rd ed. Philadelphia: Saunders, 1967, p. 922.

Page 47–Historically, there have been fewer than thirty cases per year. Kramer, Barry. "Vinyl Chloride Risks Were Known by Many Before First Deaths," *Wall Street Journal,* October 2, 1974, pp. 1 and 17.

Pages 54–55 West, Randy. "'Pete' Gettelfinger Buried Saturday at New Middletown," *The Corydon Democrat,* March 19, 1975, p. 1.

Chapter 4 Human Test Animals

Pages 57–58 In 1970, in Bologna, Dr. Cesare Maltoni began a series of experiments. Kramer, Barry. "Vinyl Chloride Risks Were Known by Many Before First Deaths," *Wall Street Journal,* October 2, 1974.

Pages 57–58 To carry out his experiments. Petition to Alexander M. Schmidt, Commissioner of the Food and Drug Administration, calling for the discontinuation of vinyl chloride and polyvinyl chloride usage in certain cosmetics and consumer products, Health Research Group, Washington, D.C., February 21, 1974, p. 6.

Page 58–liver cancer at a rate more than sixteen times normal. Testimony and slide presentation by Dr. Joseph K. Wagoner before a hearing of the California State Senate Committee on Health and Welfare, Los Angeles, California, October 23, 1975.

Page 59–carcinogenesis bioassays date back. Shimkin, M. B., and Triolo, V. A. "History of Chemical Carcinogenesis: Some Prospective Remarks," the International Symposium on Carcinogenesis and Carcinogen Testing, Boston, Massachusetts, 1967, *Progress in Experimental Tumor Research,* vol. 11, pp. 1–20, 1969.

Page 59–the essentials of the case in 1972. Saffiotti, Umberto. "The Laboratory Approach to the Identification of Environmental Carcinogens," in *Proceedings of the Ninth Canadian Cancer Research Conference,* edited by P. G. Scholefield, vol. 9, Toronto: University of Toronto Press, 1972, pp. 23 and 26–27.

Page 61–the human experience may prove far *worse* than the animal experience. Epstein, Samuel S. "The Delaney Amendment," *Preventive Medicine* 2 (March, 1973): 140–149.

Page 61–"although the direct demonstration is lacking in man." Saffiotti, Umberto. "The Laboratory Approach to the Identification of Environmental Carcinogens," pp. 26–29.

Page 62–chemical industry sales that exceeded $72 *billion*. Buder, Nancy, and Billings, Linda. "TOX-IC! Legislation to Control Toxic Substances," *Sierra Club Bulletin* (November/December, 1975): 25–27, 30–31.

Page 63–In 1940, promoters of 2-FAA. Shimkin and Triolo, "History of Chemical Carcinogenesis," pp. 11–12.

Page 63–value of carcinogenesis bioassays emerged in 1969. Innes, J. R. M., and Bates, R. R., et al. "Bioassay of Pesticides and Industrial Chemicals for Tumorigenicity in Mice: A Preliminary Note," *Journal of the National Cancer Institute* 42 (1969): 1101–1114.

Page 65–Congress heard a report. Statement of Dr. Joseph K. Wagoner before the Subcommittee on the Environment of the U.S., Senate Commerce Committee, August 21, 1974.

Page 67–urgent studies left undone. Author's communications with NIOSH officials.

Page 68–as little as 1 ppm. "Standard for Exposure to Vinyl Chloride," *Federal Register* 39 (October 4, 1974): 35890–35898.

Page 68–Despite the industry's protests and dire predictions. Mossberg, Walter. "Plastics Industry Mobilizes to Thwart Rules on Handling Vinyl Chloride," *Wall Street Journal*, June 25, 1974, p. 40.

Page 68–less than 50 ppm. Kramer, "Vinyl Chloride Risks."

Page 70–management was pressing workers to reduce vinyl chloride gas leaks. Author's interview with Pete Gettelfinger.

Page 70–began to switch from vinyl chloride. Author's communications with NIOSH officials.

Page 70–industry's representatives held the information in strictest secrecy. Polite, Dennis. "2 Groups Differ on Availability of Knowledge About Vinyl Dangers," *Louisville Times*, May 28, 1974, p. B6.

Page 70–as though there were nothing to fear. Kuttner, Bob. "Vinyl Chloride Link to Cancer Known in 1971, Report Says," *Washington Post*, September 5, 1974, p. A2.

Chapter 5 Dr. Peter Capurro

Pages 75–78 Jury, Mark. "Living in Providence Valley, Maryland Can Kill You." *Today's Health* (June 1975): 24–27, 50–52.

Pages 75–78 Buder, Nancy. "Of Poison, Man, and Indifference to Life," *Sierra Club Bulletin* (November/December 1974): 12–15.

Page 79–a fairly comprehensive list of the chemical solvents present. Capurro, Pietro U. "Effects of Chronic Exposure to Solvents

Caused by Air Pollution," *Clinical Toxicology* 3: 233–248.

Page 81–A cancer death rate "about five times higher than it should have been." "Ordeal of Providence Valley," *Medical World News* June 21, 1974.

Page 81–The chance that so many lymphomas would randomly occur. Letter to Dr. Capurro from Dr. N. E. Day, Biostatistician, International Agency for Research on Cancer, World Health Organization, February 27, 1974.

Page 81–a National Cancer Institute study. Li, Frederick P., et al. "Cancer Mortality Among Chemists," *Journal of the National Cancer Institute* 43 (November 1969): 1159–1164.

Page 82–the cause of the elevated incidence of cancer. Richards, Bill. "Cancer Rate Found High Near Md. Chemical Plant," *Washington Post*, August 12, 1974, pp. A1–A2.

Page 86 has written several scientific papers. Capurro, Peter. "Physicians, Pollution, and People," *Medical Tribune* (May 12, 1971): 4; Capurro, Pietro U. "Effects of Exposure to Solvents Caused by Air Pollution with Special Reference to CC14 and Its Distribution in Air," *Clinical Toxicology* 6 (1973): 109–124.

Chapter 6 Beyond the Factory Gates

Page 89–The State of Maryland was finally moved to conduct a study. "Interim Report: Little Elk Valley Task Force," Epidemiology and Health Effects Subcommittee, State of Maryland Department of Health and Mental Hygiene, October 28, 1975.

Page 90–"a full evaluation sometime in the future." Richards, B. "Cancer Rate Found High Near Md. Chemical Plant," *Washington Post*, August 12, 1974, pp. A1–A2.

Page 92–The Connecticut Tumor Registry reported two recent cases. U.S. Department of Health, Education and Welfare, "Epidemiologic Notes and Reports: Angiosarcoma of the Liver — Connecticut," *Morbidity and Mortality Weekly Report*, Center for Disease Control (CDC 74-8017), June 15, 1974, pp. 210 and 216.

Page 92–One case involved a woman. Brody, Jane E. "Cancer Found in Asbestos Workers' Kin," *New York Times*, September 19, 1974, pp. 1 and 27.

Page 93–Dr. Muriel L. Newhouse contributed important evidence. Brodeur, Paul. *Expendable Americans*. New York: Viking, 1974, pp. 15–16.

Page 93–sixteen common anatomic sites of the disease. U.S. Department of Health, Education and Welfare, *Atlas of Cancer Mortality for U.S. Counties: 1950-1969* (see also accompanying June 1975 "Fact Sheet"), Epidemiology Branch, National Cancer Institute (NIH 75-780).

Page 93–Inorganic arsenic. U.S. Department of Health, Education and Welfare, *Criteria for a Recommended Standard: Occupational Exposure to Inorganic Arsenic, New Criteria — 1975*, National Institute for Occupational Safety and Health (NIOSH 75-149), 1975.

Page 93–the data demonstrate above average lung cancer rates. Blot, William J., and Fraumeni, Joseph F., Jr. "Arsenical Air Pollution and Lung Cancer," *The Lancet* (July 26, 1975): 142–144.

Page 94–the mounting statistical data. Hoover, Robert, and Fraumeni, Joseph F., Jr. "Cancer Mortality in U.S. Counties with Chemical Industries," *Environmental Research* 9 (1975): 196–207.

Page 94–A study of Los Angeles. Menck, Herman R., et al. "Industrial Air Pollution: Possible Effect on Lung Cancer," *Science* 183 (January 18, 1974): 210–211.

Page 94–a similar study on Staten Island. Greenburg, Leonard, et al. "Air Pollution and Cancer Mortality: Study on Staten Island (Borough of Richmond), New York," *Archives of Environmental Health* 15 (September 1967): 356–361.

Page 94–greater than the statewide lung cancer rate. "U.S. Cancer Mortality by County," provided to author upon request by NIOSH officials.

Page 94–more than 35 percent of the people who had lived in the same house with an asbestos worker. "Asbestos Disease Spreads to Workers' Families," *Monitor*, Labor Occupational Health Program, 2 (August-September, 1975): 7.

Page 95–released the results of a major study. "The Implications of Cancer-Causing Substances in Mississippi River Water," Environmental Defense Fund, Washington, D.C., November 6, 1974.

Page 95–the General Electric Company acknowledged. "U.S. Said to Ignore a Chemical Pact," *New York Times*, January 17, 1976, p. 10.

Page 95–lengthening list of waterborne carcinogens. Hueper, Wilhelm C., and Conway, W. D. *Chemical Carcinogenesis and Cancers*. Springfield, Ill.: Thomas, 1964, pp. 688–706.

Page 96–Substantially higher mortality rates. *The Implications of Cancer-Causing Substances in Mississippi River Drinking Water*, p. 30.

Page 97–widespread cancer peril. U.S. Department of Health, Education and Welfare, "More Warnings! Vinyl Chloride — Food & Drug Administration," *Consumer News*, Office of Consumer Affairs, June 15, 1974, p. 3.

Page 97–aerosol spray cans. Buder, Nancy, and Billings, Linda. "TOX-IC! Legislation to Control Toxic Substances," *Sierra Club Bulletin* (November/December 1975): 25–27, 30–31.

Page 97–hair sprays. U.S. Department of Health, Education and Welfare, "Warnings! Hair Sprays — Food & Drug Administration," *Consumer News*, Office of Consumer Affairs, July 15, 1974, p. 3.

Page 97–indoor and outdoor pesticides. U.S. Department of

Health, Education and Welfare, "Warnings! Pesticides — Environmental Protection Agency," *Consumer News*, Office of Consumer Affairs, August 1, 1974, p. 8.

Page 98–A hospital stay generally averages. Cutler, Sidney J., et al. "Third National Cancer Survey — An Overview of Available Information," *Journal of the National Cancer Institute* 53 (December 1974): 1565–1575.

Page 98–from $5000 to $20,000. Epstein, Samuel S. "Environmental Determinants of Human Cancer," *Cancer Research* 34 (1974): 2425–2435.

Chapter 7 Ruth Beaver

Pages 103–115 Author's interviews with Ruth Beaver.

Page 105–Reprints of cigarette advertisements provided by Dr. Michael Shimkin.

Page 107–"less tars in the smoke than ever before." *Trade Regulation Rule for the Prevention of Unfair or Deceptive Advertising and Labeling of Cigarettes in Relation to the Health Hazards of Smoking, and Accompanying Statement of Basis and Purpose of Rule*, Federal Trade Commission, June 22, 1964, p. 61.

Chapter 8 Cancer for Sale

Page 116–More than 90 percent of lung cancer victims. *'76 Cancer Facts and Figures*, p. 6.

Page 116–Tar consists of hundreds of separate chemicals. U.S. Department of Health, Education and Welfare, *Smoking and Health: Report of the Advisory Committee to the Surgeon General of the Public Health Service*, 1964.

Page 116–Recent research in immunology. "Harnessing the Immunity System: from Potential to Reality" (an interview with Dr. Albert A. Good), *Ca — A Journal for Physicians*, 25 (July/August 1975): 178–186.

Page 117–If they had not smoked, at least 80 percent. *'76 Cancer Facts and Figures*, p. 5.

Page 118–"extremely rare condition." Ochsner, Alton, "Corner of History: My First Recognition of the Relationship of Smoking and Lung Cancer," *Preventive Medicine* 2 (1973): 611–614.

Page 119–Reprints of cigarette advertisements provided by Dr. Michael Shimkin.

Page 119–cigarette advertisers spent $13.8 million. *Trade Regulation Rule for the Prevention of Unfair or Deceptive Advertising and Labeling of Cigarettes in Relation to the Health Hazards of Smoking, and Accompanying*

Statement of Basis and Purpose of Rule, Federal Trade Commission, June 22, 1964, p. 71.

Page 119–cigarette advertising increased, reaching an estimated $50 million. Author's communication with Emerson Foote, cofounder of the advertising agency, Foote, Cone, and Belding.

Page 119–per capita consumption reached 690 cigarettes. U.S. Department of Agriculture, *Annual Report on Tobacco Statistics: 1942*, December, 1942, p. 82.

Page 119–the figure was 1828 cigarettes. U.S. Department of Agriculture, *Annual Report on Tobacco Statistics: 1960*, April, 1961, p. 52.

Page 120–lung cancer deaths. "United States Lung Cancer Deaths by Sex, 1930-1972," Research Department, American Cancer Society, New York, 1975.

Page 120–the first American study. Ochsner, Alton, and DeBakey, Michael. "Carcinoma of the Lung," *Archives of Surgery* 42 (February 1941): 209–258.

Page 121–"Ernst Wynder." Ochsner, "Corner of History."

Page 121–epidemiological study. Wynder, Ernest L., and Graham, Evarts A. "Tobacco Smoking as a Possible Etiologic Factor in Bronchiogenic Carcinoma: A Study of Six Hundred and Eighty-Four Proved Cases," *Journal of the American Medical Association* 143 (May 27, 1950): 329–336.

Page 122–"too much damage had been done." Ochsner, "Corner of History."

Page 122–23,502 victims. "United States Lung Cancer Deaths by Sex," American Cancer Society.

Page 122–3562 cigarettes. *Annual Report on Tobacco Statistics: 1960*, p. 52.

Page 122–over $100 million per year. *Trade Regulation Rule and Accompanying Statement*, pp. 25–76.

Page 122–an article. Norr, Roy. "Cancer by the Carton," *Reader's Digest* (December 1952): 7–8.

Page 123–television advertising in 1957. *Trade Regulation Rule and Accompanying Statement*, p. 44.

Page 123–Reprints of cigarette advertising provided by Dr. Michael Shimkin.

Page 123–"just what the doctor ordered." Wagner, Susan. *Cigarette Country: Tobacco in American History and Politics*. New York: Praeger, 1971, p. 83.

Page 123–The most influential study. Hammond, Cuyler E., and Horn, Daniel. "Smoking and Death Rates — Report on Forty-Four Months of Follow-Up of 187,783 Men (I. Total Mortality)," *Journal of the American Medical Association* 166 (March 8, 1958): 1159–1172; Hammond, Cuyler E., and Horn, Daniel. "Smoking and Death Rates —

Report on Forty-Four Months of Follow-Up of 187,783 Men (II. Death Rates by Cause)," 166 (March 15, 1958): 1294–1308.

Page 124–38,929 Americans died. "United States Lung Cancer Deaths by Sex," American Cancer Society.

Page 124–$200 million per year. *Trade Regulation Rule and Accompanying Statement*, p. 42.

Page 124–over $249 million. *Statistical Supplement to Federal Trade Commission Report to Congress Pursuant to the Public Health Cigarette Smoking Act*, December 31, 1974, p. 10.

Page 124–Surgeon General's definitive study. "Smoking and Health: Report of the Advisory Committee."

Page 125–5163 women. "United States Lung Cancer Deaths by Sex," American Cancer Society.

Page 125–incriminating data. U.S. Department of Health, Education and Welfare, *The Health Consequences of Smoking*, 1973.

Page 125–*ninety-two* times. Selikoff, Irving J., et al. "Asbestos Exposure, Smoking, and Neoplasia." *Journal of the American Medical Association* 204 (1968): 106–112.

Page 126–decline in cigarette sales of nearly 20 percent. *Statistical Supplement to Federal Trade Commission Report*, 1974, p. 4.

Page 126–"record levels of advertising." Wagner, *Cigarette Country*, p. 136.

Page 126–increased television advertising. *Statistical Supplement to Federal Trade Commission Report*, 1974, p. 10.

Page 127–agricultural and marketing subsidies. Author's communications with U.S. Department of Agriculture officials.

Page 127–one of the following warnings. *Trade Regulation Rule and Accompanying Statement*, Appendix D, p. 22.

Page 128–$261 million. *Statistical Supplement to Federal Trade Commission Report*, 1974, p. 10.

Page 128–Congress dutifully responded. "Health Warning Required on Cigarette Packs," *Congressional Quarterly Almanac* (1965): 344–351.

Page 129–per capita consumption increased in 1966. U.S. Department of Agriculture, *Annual Report on Tobacco Statistics: 1973*, April, 1974, p. 33.

Page 130–"by the tobacco companies." Terris, Milton. "A Social Policy for Health," *American Journal of Public Health* (January 1968): 5–12.

Page 130–In a landmark decision. "Applicability of the Fairness Doctrine to Cigarette Advertising," 9 F.C.C. 2d 921 (1967).

Page 130–Affirmed by the courts in 1968. *Banzhaf v. FCC*, 405 F.2d 1082 (1968).

Page 130–for every five procigarette messages. "National Broadcasting Co., Inc.," 16 F.C.C. 2d 947 (1969).

Page 130–creative anticigarette messages. Whiteside, Thomas. *Selling Death: Cigarette Advertising and Public Health.* New York: Liveright, 1971, pp. 69–71.

Page 131–major impact on cigarette consumption. *Annual Report on Tobacco Statistics: 1973*, p. 33.

Page 132–Congress intervened. "House and Senate Disagree on Cigarette Ad Bill," *Congressional Quarterly Almanac* (1969): 883–890.

Page 133–Privately, they actually favored. Gunther, Max. "Do Commercials Really *Sell* You?" *TV Guide* (November 9, 1974): 8.

Page 133–as dramatic as it was predictable. Hamilton, James L. "The Demand for Cigarettes: Advertising, the Health Scare, and the Cigarette Advertising Ban," *The Review of Economics and Statistics* (November 1972): 401–411.

Page 133–4037. *Annual Report on Tobacco Statistics: 1973*, p. 33.

Page 133–4147. U.S. Department of Agriculture, *Annual Report on Tobacco Statistics: 1975*, April 1976, p. 28.

Page 133–advised Congress to allocate funds. *Federal Trade Commission Report to Congress Pursuant to the Public Health Cigarette Smoking Act*, December 31, 1974, pp. 10–11.

Page 135–about $50 million annually. U.S. Department of Agriculture, "Costs of Selected Items on Tobacco for Fiscal Years 1970–1975, and Estimates for 1976–1977," March 12, 1976.

Page 136–theory and actual studies. "Low Tar, Nicotine Cigarettes Cut Death Rate, Cancer Society Says," *Los Angeles Times*, September 15, 1976, Part I, p. 11.

Page 137–several hundred thousand small tobacco farmers. U.S. Department of Agriculture, "Tobacco in the National Economy," 1975.

Page 138–surveys indicate that even among smokers themselves. "Gallop Poll Index," commissioned by the American Cancer Society, New York, June, 1974.

Page 139–cancer mortality among Mormons. Lyon, Joseph L., et al. "Cancer Incidence in Mormons and Non-Mormons in Utah, 1966–1970," *New England Journal of Medicine* 294 (January 15, 1976): 129–133; Enstrom, James E. "Cancer Mortality Among Mormons," *Cancer* 36 (September 1975): 825–841.

Page 139–even more so by heavy drinking. "Heavy Drinking Adds to the Risk of Cancers of Mouth and Throat," *Journal of the American Medical Association* 229 (August 19, 1974): 1023–1024.

Page 139–occurring 66 percent less. Lyon, et al. "Cancer Incidence in Mormons and Non-Mormons," p. 132.

Page 139–Among women, these malignancies kill more than 25,000. *'76 Cancer Facts and Figures*, p. 9.

Page 139–recent evidence indicating that the standard American diet. Howell, Margaret A. "Diet as an Etiological Factor in the Development of Cancers of the Colon and Rectum," *Journal of Chronic Diseases* 28 (February 1975): 67–80; Burkitt, Denis P. "Epidemiology of Cancer of the Colon and Rectum." *Cancer* 28 (1971): 3–13; Weisburger, J. H. "Environmental Cancer," *Journal of Occupational Medicine* 18 (April 1976): 245–252.

Page 140–are prone to endometrial cancer. Garnet, James D. "Constitutional Stigmas Associated with Endometrial Carcinoma," *American Journal of Obstetrics and Gynecology* (July 1958): 11–19.

Page 140–increase in uterine cancer. Smith, Donald C., et al. "Association of Exogenous Estrogen and Endometrial Carcinoma," *The New England Journal of Medicine* 293 (December 4, 1975): 1164–1170.

Page 140–about $80 million annually. "Estrogen Is Linked to Uterine Cancer," *New York Times*, December 4, 1975, pp. 1 and 55.

Page 140–reported their observations. Mays, E. Truman, et al. "Hepatic Changes in Young Women Ingesting Contraceptive Steroids," *Journal of the American Medical Association* 235 (February 16, 1976): 730–732.

Page 141–a recent California study. Fasal, Elfriede, and Paffenbarger, Ralph S., Jr. "Oral Contraceptives as Related to Cancer and Benign Lesions of the Breast," *Journal of the National Cancer Institute* 55 (October 1975): 767–773.

Chapter 9 Jennie Day

Pages 145–154 Author's interviews with Polly and Julian Day.

Chapter 10 Childhood Cancers

Page 155–more than 6000 new cases. *'76 Cancer Facts and Figures*, pp. 13 and 22.

Page 155–A recent review. Pratt, Charles B., et al. "'Adult Type' Cancer in Children and Adolescents," St. Jude Children's Research Hospital, Memphis, Tennessee, 1976.

Page 156–can have a considerably shorter latent period. Hueper, *Chemical Carcinogenesis*, p. 43.

Page 156–nearly half of the radiation exposure. *Effects of Chronic Exposure to Low-Level Pollutants in the Environment*, prepared by the Congressional Research Service for the Subcommittee on the Environment and the Atmosphere of the Committee on Science and Technology, U.S. House of Representatives, 94th Cong., 1st Sess., November, 1975, pp. 35–41.

Page 157–triggering a malignancy. Favus, Murray J., et al. "Thyroid Cancer Occurring as a Late Consequence of Head-and-Neck

Irradiation," *The New England Journal of Medicine* 294 (May 6, 1976): 1019–1025; Spiegelhalter, Joan. "Radiation Exposure Is Real Problem to Women," *Clip Sheet*, University of California at Berkeley, July 21, 1975.

Page 157–According to Selikoff. Burros, Marian. "Asbestos Found in Baby Powders," *Los Angeles Times*, March 8, 1976, Part I, p. 1.

Page 157–its uses are myriad. Blejer, Hector P., and Arlon, Robert. "Talc: A Possible Occupational and Environmental Carcinogen," *Journal of Occupational Medicine* 15 (February 1973): 92–97.

Page 158–is coated with glucose and talc. "Rice," *Consumer Reports* (July 1976): 376–377.

Page 158–Nitrate and nitrite are used. Jacobson, Michael F. *Eater's Digest: The Consumer's Factbook of Food Additives*. Garden City, New York: Doubleday, 1972, pp. 164–170.

Page 158–nitrosamines are powerful carcinogens. Lijinsky, William, and Epstein, Samuel S. "Nitrosamines as Environmental Carcinogens," *Nature* 225 (January 3, 1970): 21–23.

Page 159–a food-linked nitrosamine cancer toll. Jacobson, Michael F., *"Don't Bring Home the Bacon": How Sodium Nitrite Can Affect Your Health*. Washington, D.C.: Center for Science in the Public Interest, March, 1973.

Page 159–afflicted with liver tumors. Petition to Alexander M. Schmidt, Commissioner of the Food and Drug Administration, Health Research Group, pp. 6–7.

Page 160–In increasing numbers, women. U.S. Department of Health, Education and Welfare, Hunt, Vilma R. *Occupational Health Problems of Pregnant Women: A Report and Recommendations for the Office of the Secretary*, April 30, 1975.

Page 160–Dr. Michael Shimkin and others. Shimkin, Michael B., et al. "Induction of Testicular Tumors and Other Effects of Stilbestrol-Cholesterol Pellets in Strain C Mice," *Journal of the National Cancer Institute* 2 (1941): 65–80.

Page 161–but in their female children. Benton, Barbara D. A. "Stilbestrol and Vaginal Cancer," *American Journal of Nursing* (May 1974): 900–901; Brozan, Nadine. "Repercussions of a Drug: An Ordeal for Mothers and Their Daughters — and Maybe Their Sons," *New York Times*, June 17, 1976, p. 41.

Page 161–Rachel Carson included a chapter. Carson, Rachel. *Silent Spring*. Boston: Houghton Mifflin, 1962, pp. 22, 195–216.

Page 162–halt the use of aldrin and dieldrin. "Shell Chemical Co. et al.: Consolidated Aldrin/Dieldrin Hearing," *Federal Register* 39 (October 18, 1974): 37216–37272.

Page 164–"producing malignant tumors." "Notice of Intent to Cancel Registrations of Certain Pesticide Products Containing Heptachlor or Chlordane," Environmental Protection Agency, November 18, 1974.

Page 164–epidemiologists today. Author's communications with NIOSH officials.

Page 164–Kepone as the latest carcinogenic pesticide. Dunford, Earle. "Kepone: Center of Environmental Furor," *National Observer*, January 10, 1976, p. 6.

Page 165–The results released. U.S. Department of Health, Education and Welfare, "Report on Carcinogenesis Bioassay of Technical Grade Chlordecone (Kepone)," National Cancer Institute, National Institutes of Health, April 8, 1976.

Page 165–recommended reduced reliance on chlorinated hydrocarbon pesticides. "Use of Pesticides: A Report of the President's Advisory Committee," The White House, May 15, 1963.

Page 165–a similar recommendation. U.S. Department of Health, Education and Welfare, *Report of the Secretary's Commission on Pesticides and Their Relationship to Environmental Health, Parts I and II*, December, 1969.

Page 166–evidence of their carcinogenecity. *IARC Monographs on the Evaluation of Carcinogenic Risk of Chemicals to Man: Some Organochlorine Pesticides*, vol. 5. International Agency for Research on Cancer, 1974.

Page 166–remain in widespread use. Author's communications with EPA officials.

Page 166–two Canadian investigators. Fabia, Jacqueline, and Thuy, Truong Dam. "Occupation of Father at Time of Birth of Children Dying of Malignant Diseases," *British Journal of Preventive Social Medicine* 28 (1974): 98–100.

Page 167–miscarriages or giving birth to stillborn infants. "Vinyl Chloride Linked to Fetal Deaths," *Los Angeles Times*, February 4, 1976, Part I, p. 4.

Page 167–excessive numbers of chromosomal breaks. U.S. Department of Health, Education and Welfare, Infante, Peter F., et al. "Genetic Risks of Vinyl Chloride," Division of Field Studies and Clinical Investigations, National Institute for Occupational Safety and Health, November 17, 1975.

Page 167–data from a 1975 Ohio Study. U.S. Department of Health, Education and Welfare, "Epidemiologic Notes and Reports: Vinyl Chloride and Congenital Malformations — Ohio," *Morbidity and Mortality Weekly Report* (for week ending July 19, 1975), Center for Disease Control, vol. 24, July 25, 1975, pp. 245–246.

Chapter 11 Dr. Wilhelm Hueper

Page 171–Dr. Epstein began his remarks. Presentation by Dr. Samuel S. Epstein of the First Annual Award of the Society for Occupational and Environmental Health to Dr. Wilhelm C. Hueper, New York City, March 25, 1975.

Pages 171–186 Author's interviews with Dr. Hueper.
Page 176–finally succeeded in 1938. Hueper, Wilhelm C., et al. "Experimental Production of Bladder Tumors in Dogs by Administration of Beta-naphthylamine," *Journal of Industrial Hygiene* 20 (1938): 46–84.
Page 176–grim vindication came. Auerbach, Stuart. "N.J.'s Chemical Belt Takes Its Toll," *Washington Post*, February 8, 1976, pp. A1–A2.
Page 177–"the new artificial environment." Hueper, Wilhelm C. *Occupational Tumors and Allied Diseases*. Springfield, Ill.: Thomas, 1942, pp. 3–10.
Pages 180–181 Testimony of Dr. Wilhelm C. Hueper before the House Select Committee to Investigate the Use of Chemicals in Foods and Cosmetics, House of Representatives, 82nd Cong., 2nd Sess., Part 3, 1952, pp. 1353–1382.
Page 181–questioned the safety of Red Dye No. 2. Franks, Lucinda. "Red Dye No. 2: The 20-Year Battle," *New York Times*, February 28, 1976, p. 20; Boffey, Philip M. "Death of a Dye?" *New York Times Magazine*, February 29, 1976, pp. 9 and 48–51.
Page 185–carcinogenic contaminants in cosmetics. Hueper, Wilhelm C., and Conway, W. D. *Chemical Carcinogenesis and Cancers*. Springfield, Ill.: Thomas, 1964, pp. 676–684.
Page 186–"the majority of human cancer is potentially preventable." World Health Organization, *Prevention of Cancer* (WHO technical Report Series No. 276), p. 4.

Chapter 12 Toward a New Ethic

Page 187–classical trilogy. Hueper, Wilhelm C., and Conway, W. D. *Chemical Carcinogenesis and Cancers*. Springfield, Ill.: Thomas, 1964; Hueper, Wilhelm C., *Occupational and Environmental Cancers of the Respiratory Tract*, vol. 3, *Recent Results in Cancer Research*. New York: Springer-Verlag, 1966; Hueper, Wilhelm C., *Occupational and Environmental Cancers of the Urinary System*. New Haven, Connecticut: Yale University Press, 1969.
Page 188–outlawed the manufacture and use of benzidine. Wagoner, Joseph K. "Occupational Carcinogenesis: The Two Hundred Years Since Percivall Pott," in Saffiotti, Umberto, and Wagoner, Joseph K., eds. *Annals of the New York Academy of Sciences: Occupational Carcinogenesis*, vol. 271, New York: The New York Academy of Sciences, 1976, pp. 1–4.
Page 188–high school and college students. "Carcinogen Survey in California Schools," California State Department of Health, March, 1976.
Page 188–Gerald Ford's presidential order. "Ford Drives to Gut

OSHA," *Spotlight on Health and Safety*, Industrial Union Department, AFL-CIO, vol. 5, no. 2, 1976, pp. 1–2.

Page 188–Dr. Hueper urged. Hueper, *Chemical Carcinogenesis*, pp. 624–626.

Page 189–federal officials investigating a plant in Georgia. Wagoner, "Occupational Carcinogenesis: The Two Hundred Years Since Percivall Pott."

Page 190–"rendering an accounting for such acts." Hueper, *Chemical Carcinogenesis*, p. 634.

Page 190–The solution he believed. Author's interviews with Dr. Hueper.

Page 192–less than 20 percent. Address of Congressman David R. Obey before the Society for Occupational and Environmental Health, December, 1974; "NCI Reports $120 Million — 17% of Budget — for Env. Carcinogenesis," *The Cancer Letter*, February 20, 1976, pp. 4–8.

Page 194–a 50 percent overall improvement. Author's communications with Dr. Hueper.

Page 194–Other estimates. Schneiderman, Marvin A. "Environmental Factors and Cancer Prevention," Field Studies and Statistics Program, Division of Cancer Cause and Prevention, National Cancer Institute, 1976; Brody, Jane E. "Cancer Control a Fight on 100 Diseases," *New York Times*, December 9, 1975, pp. 1 and 23.

Page 195–Dr. Umberto Saffiotti described. Author's interview with Dr. Saffiotti.

Page 196–"That is my testament." Author's interview with Dr. Hueper.

Index